THE
HEALER
WITHIN

My Recovery from Chronic Lyme, CFS, And Autoimmune Disease

HOLLY L. CHAMELI

Copyright 2019. All Rights Reserved.

No part of this publication may be reproduced, distributed, or transmitted in any form or by any means, including photocopying, recording, or other electronic or mechanical methods, or by any information storage and retrieval system without the prior written permission of the publisher, except in the case of very brief quotations embodied in critical reviews and certain other noncommercial uses permitted by copyright law.

FOR MORE INFORMATION VISIT: thehealerwithin.me

Disclaimer

I am not a medical professional, nor do I have any formal training in nutrition, medicine, or healing. The advice and information contained in this book are solely based on my personal experiences and opinions from living with and naturally treating Lyme disease, autoimmune disease, and chronic fatigue syndrome. While I have heavily cited sources in the endnotes at the end of the book, there are many times in which I am writing from memory from my own personal research and the many hours spent consulting with medical doctors, naturopaths, functional medicine practitioners, acupuncturists, certified nutritionists, and others. Although I have made every effort to ensure the information in this book is well cited, accurate, and correct, I do not assume and hereby disclaim any liability to any party for any loss, damage, or disruption caused by errors or omissions, whether such errors or omissions result from negligence, accident, or any other cause.

Throughout the book, I sometimes quote or refer to other medical professionals who I either sought treatment from directly or whose book(s) I used as points of reference for my treatment. These medical professionals did not endorse this book, and the opinions expressed in this book are not necessarily shared by these practitioners. Any quoted material from medical professionals or others in this book are limited and protected by the fair use doctrine.

Also note, throughout this book I frequently refer to Lyme disease that has gone either untreated or unresolved for more than a year as "chronic Lyme disease." Please know that "chronic Lyme disease" is a controversial diagnosis. Most medical doctors do not recognize it, and may instead diagnose a patient with post-treatment Lyme disease syndrome (PLDS)[1] should symptoms not resolve with a few weeks of antibiotics. I fail to personally believe in PLDS, however, so I use the term "chronic Lyme disease."

The advice contained herein is not medical advice and should be fully reviewed by your medical doctor before implementing. This book is not intended to diagnose or treat any illness or condition. The reader should regularly consult a medical doctor in matters relating to his or her health, particularly with respect to any symptoms that may require diagnosis or medical treatment.

CONTENTS

Preface vii

PART I:
MY STORY & AN INTRODUCTION TO CHRONIC ILLNESS

Chapter 1   My Story..7
Chapter 2   My Story—Part II 21
Chapter 3   Understanding Mystery Illnesses—
                     Lyme Disease, Chronic Fatigue Syndrome ("CFS"),
                     Fibromyalgia & Autoimmune Disease 29
Chapter 4   Coming To Terms 39

PART II:
THE HEAVY LIFTING OF GETTING WELL

Chapter 5   A Crash Course in Gut Health &
                     Your Roadmap to Health..49
Chapter 6   RECOVERY STEP #1—Implement a Targeted
                     & Nutrient-Dense Diet..54
Chapter 7   RECOVERY STEP #2—Balance Your Hormones......68
Chapter 8   RECOVERY STEP #3—Combat Infection with
                     Targeted Herbal Protocols..83
Chapter 9   RECOVERY STEP #4—Restore Proper Balance
                     to Your Microbiome...104
Chapter 10   RECOVERY STEP #5—Implement Gentle
                     Detox & Support Modalities 108

Chapter 11 RECOVERY STEP #6—Restore Energy with
            Targeted Nutrition, Exercise, and Supplementation ... 114
Chapter 12 RECOVERY STEP #7—Detoxify Your
            Environment..129
Chapter 13 RECOVERY STEP #8—Implement Effective
            Coping & Stress Management Strategies 141
Chapter 14 Finding A Practitoner & Reliable Resources............... 157
Chapter 15 Final Words... 163

Endnotes 171

For their love and support, this book is dedicated to my mom and dad, my husband Paul, and my two children, Emma & JP.

PREFACE

"The wound is the place where the light enters you."
Rumi

In January 2012, I fell sick with a mysterious and chronic illness for which there was no cure. Up to that point in time, I'd been an otherwise active and healthy, 36 year-old mother of two who regularly ran four miles per day with my kids in a double jogger. I watched my diet and was never overweight. But regardless, just a few months after the birth of my second child, and literally overnight, I became acutely ill with a condition doctors could not diagnose. Ultimately, I required so much care that I landed at my parents' house, hours away from my husband with my infant children in tow.

I was bedridden for about two years and disabled for the better part of a decade. I lived with my parents for the first 4 ½ years of this nightmare, relying upon them for almost everything. I went from doctor to doctor, desperate for a diagnosis or some semblance of an explanation as to what was wrong with my body. I took antibiotics, IVs of ozone and vitamins, tons of supplements, followed special diets and herbal treatments, sought advice from all sorts of medical practitioners—from the top medical doctors at the Cleveland Clinic to naturopaths, functional medicine practitioners, acupuncturists, certified nutritionists, on and on. I left no stone unturned in my quest for health. My symptoms ranged from chronic, bone-crushing fatigue to joint pain, insomnia, and body tremors, to name just a few.

Over the course of several years, I was diagnosed with Lyme disease, chronic fatigue syndrome ("CFS"), fibromyalgia, Hashimoto's thyroiditis, and a few other autoimmune conditions, and was also told by a doctor that I had "nothing wrong" and was encouraged to go home and "walk it off." Hard to walk something off when you cannot walk more than 25 yards. Sadly, medical doctors did almost nothing for me, except take my money and make me more sick by offering prescriptions of antibiotics, steroids, pain medication, and sleeping pills.

Out of sheer desperation to get well, I gave up on traditional medical doctors and turned my attention to holistic and functional medicine. Eventually, by following the principles outlined in this book, I found my way back to health.

But it was *not* easy.

While sick and bedridden, I researched all sorts of alternative therapies and scribbled ideas on a legal notebook at my bedside. Through literal trial and error, and by essentially using my body as a science experiment, I found my way in the dark. There were days I was certain I would never be well again. In fact, I purchased my burial plot with my disability funds at one point. But deep inside, I never gave up. Every day, I put one foot in front of the other, always following my protocol and diet and trusting things would turn around. And ever so slowly, they did.

Whether you're struggling with Lyme disease, chronic fatigue syndrome, fibromyalgia, lupus, rheumatoid arthritis, or any other chronic health problem or "mystery illness," my experiences will be beneficial to your recovery. The protocols I followed and principles I adhered to (and still do) are used by functional medicine practitioners and naturopaths to treat a wide range of ailments, from cancer and MS to Lyme disease and fibromyalgia. My approach is broad in its range, but specific in that it is geared toward healing at the cellular level.

Life itself is the greatest of teachers. This experience has taught me an enormous amount about health and wellness, and now I get to share what I've learned with you. If you or a loved one is going through a chronic and debilitating illness, please keep the faith and keep moving forward. The human body is truly amazing in its capacity to heal.

We all deserve to enjoy our time on this earth in good health. I sincerely hope this book will help you on your journey to wellness.

Let's begin.

PART I

My Story & An Introduction to Chronic Illness

CHAPTER ONE

MY STORY

"There is no education like adversity."
Benjamin Disraeli

I fell sick overnight, both literally and figuratively. I liken it to being mugged, only instead of losing my wallet, I lost something much more valuable—my health. Within a 24-hour period in 2012, my world went from being an active and healthy wife and mother of two, to a life of chronic and debilitating pain and fatigue that rendered me simply unable to function. Ultimately, over the course of many months, this mysterious illness left me bedridden, living at my parents' house hours away from my husband, with two young children under the age of three. I became completely reliant upon my parents for my care. And worse, I was unable to find any competent doctor to tell me what was wrong or what to do to fix it.

The On-set

It was Friday, January 13, 2012. I had just turned 36 years old. I woke up that morning to several inches of snow in our new apartment situated outside of Detroit, Michigan. I was quite upset that the weather was going to disrupt my workout plans that morning, as I'd been planning to break-in my new double jogger stroller on a long run outdoors with the kids. I recall standing in front of my blender at breakfast, doubly agitated to find my blueberries for the morning's smoothie were gone. Being out of blueberries and angry at the weather would soon be the least of my problems; I was woefully unready for the tsunami about to derail my life.

Many people recall a "trigger" or some sort of traumatic event that brought about their symptoms. For me, I believe it was a perfect storm of stress and a common antibiotic I'd taken that morning with my breakfast. I had a very benign health issue that did not genuinely warrant an antibiotic, but the urgent care doctor the previous night gave it to me anyway. I'd also been wrestling a fair amount of stress in my personal life, trying to keep several balls in the air as a new working mother. To be blunt, I was tired and worn down.

On this particular day, however, I woke up feeling great. Later that morning, I headed out for a full day of house showings with several realtors. I was optimistic about finding us a permanent place to settle. But, fast forward five hours to the drive home, and I felt overcome by what initially seemed like the on-set of flu.

As soon as I got home, I took some aspirin. Within two hours, I was experiencing severe pain in almost every joint in my body. Even navigating the stairs was painful, as it caused shooting pains in my hip joints. I felt feverish and achy. I instinctively knew something was very wrong. This felt nothing like a typical case of the flu. In fact, it felt unlike anything I'd ever experienced to that point in my life.

That night in bed, I sweated like I was sleeping in a jungle. I had to change my night shirt twice. I got up early the next morning, and as I was explaining how sick I felt to my husband, I also realized I was seeing funny. The carpet on the floor looked fuzzier to me than normal. When I looked at the wall, it appeared to have movement to it, like small fishies everywhere. Then, I looked in the mirror and saw red dots all over my arms and chest, and eyes so bloodshot it looked like I had been drinking heavily.

I staggered back to the urgent care later that morning, very concerned I'd had an allergic reaction to my antibiotic. The doctor ran basic bloodwork, which revealed nothing. He felt I might have reacted to my medication and advised me to stop taking it. He said any allergic reaction would self-correct in a few days, and advised me to drink plenty of liquids. I went home feeling terribly sick and went to bed.

Days, then weeks, passed without improvement. I was keenly aware that no one else in our home was catching whatever it was that I'd contracted. I decided I had better find a decent doctor to help me. I scheduled an appointment with a well-regarded general practitioner for later that week.

And that's when it happened. As swiftly as this mysterious illness had swept in and enveloped me, it vanished! I woke up the day before my doctor appointment and felt entirely better—no joint pain, no body aches, no sign of fever. I was so relieved. My nightmare was over! I called the general practitioner and cancelled my appointment.

Unfortunately, my excitement would be short-lived.

The following day, "it" returned. Midway through a photoshoot for the kids at the mall, I fell feverish and achy. By the time the photoshoot ended, I felt the worst flu of my life once again taking hold.

What was going on with me? When I got home, I called the general practitioner and rescheduled my appointment.

Queue the Revolving Doctor Visits

I didn't know it at the time, but this initial visit with the general practitioner would be the first of many unproductive doctor visits for me. Looking back, it is laughable how naïve I was about medical doctors and their ability to "fix" people. All my life I'd assumed that when you got sick, you simply went to the doctor, he performed a test, diagnosed you, treated you, then sent you home to get better. While this is true for many conditions—like broken legs and sinus infections—it was not going to be the case for me. I was about to receive a serious lesson on how the medical industry works, the true meaning of healthcare, and my own role and responsibility in my personal well-being.

My visit with the general practitioner uncovered nothing wrong except high inflammation, elevated autoimmune activity, and an elevated white blood cell count. He sent me to a rheumatologist who was very well-intentioned, but was ultimately unable to provide any help. I vividly remember that first visit to the rheumatologist's office, as I was so weak and in so much pain that my husband had to assist me in walking from the car into the building. I recall sitting in the waiting room that day looking around at the other patients, wondering if they too felt as sick as I did. Is this what it felt like to have a rheumatic disease? *These poor people*, I thought.

After the rheumatologist examined me, she sat down in her chair, put her hand on her chin, and was silent for a few moments. She was perplexed. It was becoming very clear to me that this was not, in fact, what most other rheumatology patients experienced, at least not the ones this doctor treated. She sent me for an x-ray and a litany of blood tests. My blood tests showed elevated white blood cells and systemic inflammation, but nothing specific enough for a diagnosis. The doctor then offered me steroids, and said she hoped my symptoms would work themselves out over time. I was once again sent home very sick with no recourse or recommendation as to what to do.

While at home sick in bed, I became obsessed with finding answers. I began to furiously research on-line about my symptoms. Lyme disease kept popping up. I read story after story of people who either had no memory of a bulls-eye rash before falling sick, or who had developed one many years before symptoms presented.

That is when I recalled an incident from several years prior in New York State. After walking near a wooded area with my dog, I developed a very large concentric bulls-eye rash on my left bicep. I noticed it a few days after my walk as I passed a mirror in the hallway. I stopped and lifted my sleeve to reveal a perfect set of concentric rings about the size of a softball. I felt fine, but went downstairs to show my mother. She immediately suspected Lyme disease and urged me to go to the doctor. Not having any symptoms, I was not at all worried about it. I went to the doctor shortly thereafter and was told flatly, after a cursory exam without any blood testing, that I did not have Lyme disease. I recall pushing the issue with the doctor, as the bulls-eye rash made me nervous, but he brushed off my concerns. He felt the rash was fading and therefore posed no problem. Trusting the doctor, I left his office and went along with my life.

What I didn't know at that time is that Lyme disease is a very sneaky, stealth infection that can sit idle in your body lurking and waiting for the right time to explode.[2] It creates its own sheath called a biofilm where it can live for years unchecked and suppressed by the immune system until the right set of circumstances opens the floodgates into the bloodstream.[3] The biofilm that protects Lyme infections is one of many reasons it is so difficult to kill with antibiotics. The antibiotics often cannot effectively penetrate the biofilm.[4]

After reading numerous anecdotal stories on-line and recalling my bulls-eye rash in New York State, I was convinced Lyme disease was my problem. I went back to my rheumatologist and asked to be tested. The test came back negative. Back to the drawing board.

At this point, I was certain I had MS or something potentially worse like cancer. My symptoms had been on-going for months with no reprieve. Along with my original symptoms, I was now experiencing body tremors, terrible brain fog, fatigue, difficulty focusing and holding conversations, swollen lymph nodes, stabbing pains in my knees, shins and various muscles, weakness on the entire right side of my face, tingling sensations on my tongue, odd sensations on my head, neck and legs as if cold water was trickling down my skin, swelling and redness in my toes and fingers, and pain in the balls of my feet whenever I would stand.

Not having any clear-cut plan of attack or knowing what was wrong with my body, I clung to what I knew—exercise and nutrition. It had been my experience up to that point that exercise helped just about everything. My dad, an avid runner, had always told us growing up that the best thing to do if we felt sick was to go running. He'd tell us that getting our body temperature up, sweating, and increasing circulation would burn up whatever bug we'd caught.

So, I started running again—slowly. It wasn't easy. Every inch of my body ached, but regardless, I would put on my running clothes and hit the road. The first few times I went to our local park, my knees hurt so badly I was only able to run a few steps, then walk, and then repeat for a single lap. But I kept at it. How sick could I have been if I was still able to exercise? You'd be amazed. Imagine the worst flu of your life, and I hobbled through it. I found that exercise was the only thing that gave me any relief from the pain. Ten minutes into one of my slow walk-hobble-run workouts, and the aches started to ease up a bit.

After a month or so, my stamina improved, and I was noticing an overall decrease in my joint pain. Eventually, over the course of several months, I was able to run again with my kids in the jogger. By the end of my runs, I felt almost "normal," or as close to it as I could remember. I also began juicing, limiting my sugar intake, and following what I believed to be a healthy diet. I thought I was on my way to recovery. I felt if I just kept up my program, my good days would increase in number.

But unfortunately that did not happen.

Gradually, no matter how diligent my efforts, I just could not seem to get well. Feeling normal eluded me, no matter how hard I worked. I'd go a period of feeling tolerable and then at the drop of a dime, I'd be overcome with what felt like a heavy flu and severe brain fog. As the weeks went by, I tried to keep a smile on my face and maintain a positive attitude, but I knew I was falling apart. Eventually, the ten good days I had a month turned to seven, then five, and then I was right back where I had started.

Going through this with small children at home was very difficult. My children were seven months and two years old, respectively, at the time and heavily relied upon me for everything. My daughter had just recently started ballet classes, which she loved. I wanted to stay and watch her dance each week, like the other mothers did, but even this simple activity of sitting and watching her was impossible for me. I ached so badly, sitting still and having to interact with the other parents was unbearable. Instead, I would pull my car up to the fire lane in front of the building, run my daughter inside, and then go back to my car and cry. A few months after enrolling her, the ballet lessons had to stop. I was too tired and in too much pain to even get her there.

Eventually, I aligned with an infectious disease doctor who re-tested me for Lyme disease. This time, oddly, I tested positive on the CDC's western blot test. This is like hitting the lottery for a Lyme disease sufferer, because many who have the disease never test "CDC positive." So, in this sense, I was lucky.

After all I had read the past several months about Lyme disease, I knew I needed to find a doctor who specialized in it. At this point, I'd already been very sick for almost a full year without any treatment whatsoever. I wasted no time with this infectious disease doctor, as she was young and made it known she hadn't handled many Lyme cases. Instead, I found a local Lyme Literate Medical Doctor ("LLMD") and scheduled a consultation. I didn't realize at the time just how lucky I was to have a LLMD in my vicinity, as most people do not.

The LLMD re-tested me for Lyme disease and its co-infections. I tested positive once again for Lyme, and also tested positive for the co-infection babesia. The test for babesia was a PCR test that checks for the DNA of bacteria in the blood—a much more reliable test than the antiquated CDC Lyme disease test, which only detects antibodies. Babesia is a common co-infection of Lyme disease and is known to cause severe night sweats, air hunger, and bloodshot eyes, each of which had been initial primary symptoms of mine. I also had my blood stained and reviewed under a microscope. This test revealed what appeared to be giant globules in my blood, which were identified as biofilm colonies. Inside these biofilm colonies, explained my doctor, lived the organisms that were making me chronically sick. The LLMD immediately started me on antibiotics for several weeks.

From here, my health went completely off the rails and nose-dived into the ground. Within weeks of taking the antibiotics, I was bedridden, unable to do much except stagger to the kitchen and back in a foggy haze. Eventually, I had to completely give up on antibiotics. I simply could not handle them. The more I took, the closer to death I felt. Having two kids at home to care for, it quickly became nearly impossible to function. My LLMD, faced with this knowledge, could offer little help aside from a referral to a local naturopath who also specialized in Lyme disease.

In January of 2013, exhausted, sick, and terrified for my future, I began a round of alternative treatments with this recommended naturopath. Treatments consisted of herbal and homeopathic remedies and various supplements. But it all seemed too little too late. By March, I was unable to walk further than about fifty yards without needing assistance or having to sit down. Before long, it digressed into not being able to get off the bed. I needed someone to help me around the clock, as I could barely muster the energy to make my own meals. My husband, consumed with work obligations and overwhelmed by the enormity of my health problems, urged me to go home to my parents' house in New York State where we had more family and resources available.

I laid in bed, traumatized at the realization that I could no longer care for my children unassisted. I vividly recall that moment feeling like a drowning person grasping for whatever was within arm's reach to cling to for safety. My parents' home was a lifeboat in my mind, and I had to get to it.

Moving In With My Parents

I do not remember arriving at my parents' home. I just know that once I got there, my health continued to spiral downward and my family was intensely worried. I would find out a few years later that my parents had put me on the church prayer list, which is never a good sign.

Looking back, I try to put myself in my family's position. My parents were approaching 70 years old and had their daughter debilitated at their doorstep with her two young children. My husband was living five hours and four states away, having to work a very demanding job while his wife was completely bedridden. Seeing me and the kids required him to drive ten hours on weekends after a long work week. I am not sure who had it worse—me or my family. The stress on everyone was immense. And certainly no one knew what to do.

One thing I did know, though, was that I could not handle anymore antibiotics. However, I had to do something to combat whatever had taken over my body. I could not continue to lay in bed, day after day, and get worse. I consulted with my former LLMD via phone, and he recommended two types of treatment that could be performed at a local doctor's office near my parents' home. The first was intravenous ("IV") and high dose vitamin C therapy. He explained that IV vitamin C treatment was a gentler approach to antibiotics, but that the high dose administered directly into the bloodstream had the capacity to kill infection quite effectively. He also recommended IV ozone therapy. IV ozone therapy oxygenates the blood, making it less hospitable to infection.

It all sounded a little crazy to me. I'd never heard of IV vitamins or IV ozone before this point in my life, and had anyone asked me a year prior if this was something I would ever consider, I'd have looked at them cock-eyed. Growing sicker with each day, however, I felt I had little choice and nothing to lose. I researched both treatments very thoroughly before starting, and I discovered a large community of Lyme patients who attributed their recoveries to ozone or vitamin C therapy, or both. Perhaps I would be one of them, but I wouldn't know until I tried.

For the next month, my mother carted me to and from twice-weekly IV treatments. Some weeks went better than others. There were days when I could not even tolerate the car ride to the doctor's office. The visual of anything moving past the car window was stimulation overload to the point it made me very sick. Two minutes into the drive, and my mom was turning around and helping me stagger back to my bed. On the days when I was able to get through my treatments, I would walk in feeling achy, spacey, and weak, and walk out feeling even more achy, spacey, and weak. The ozone treatments, especially, made me very tired and exacerbated my symptoms. It took me days to recover, and by "recover," I mean I was once again able to get up out of bed and stagger around for an hour or two per day in my pajamas. But, I hoped from all I'd read that this was merely a "die-off reaction," which is common during Lyme disease treatment. A die-off—or "Herxheimer reaction"—occurs when the infection dies off at a faster rate than the body can handle. The dead waste can build up, especially in a person with a compromised immune system, resulting in heightened discomfort and symptoms until the waste is properly detoxed by the body.[5]

And that was my mindset through it all—blind hope and faith. I *hoped* I was, in fact, getting better. Because that is the thing with these treatments and this disease—*you never truly know anything*. You hope and wait and see. You could be experiencing a die-off reaction and actual healing, or you could just be getting more sick. That is just the way it is, like it or not. And meanwhile, as you are suffering the physical symptoms of the disease, self-doubt and what-if questions dance around in your mind. Try as you might to remain confident and steadfast in your protocol and belief you will get well, it is always hard to gauge which direction you are headed. You must develop a faith and belief in your instinctual feelings, because they are all you have to truly rely upon.

Ultimately, I completed about eight weeks of these treatments before I decided to give my body a break.

Dark Days

The emotional toll of this was heavy. On a daily basis, I feared the very worst. Every morning for the better part of a year, I spent breakfast in tears with my mother trying to console me. She would tell me, "just keep doing what you're doing, it will get better." I wasn't sure if she was right, but hearing her say it made me feel it was possible. Her words were like medicine.

Not knowing what else to do, we scheduled a series of appointments with specialists at the Cleveland Clinic. Somehow I knew even this would be a waste of time, but we just had to *do something*. Most of all, my family and I needed a highly qualified doctor to put our minds at ease that I would recover.

The Cleveland Clinic

At the Cleveland Clinic, I met with three doctors—an infectious disease doctor, an internist, and an endocrinologist—over two separate days. In retrospect, it was an outrageously expensive and counterproductive exercise in futility, wherein I once again hobbled away extremely sick with no answers.

The infectious disease doctor I met with was very personable, but offered no help. After reviewing my medical records, he summarily dismissed Lyme disease as the possible culprit, because he said I'd already taken the requisite dosage of doxycycline to kill a Lyme infection. At this point, he said the best he could do was have me go home and not consider myself a "sick person." Get lots of rest and maintain a healthy lifestyle, was his advice. He projected that I might recover in another 18 months. Why 18 months? I have no idea. It was a date plucked from the sky. Then, he ordered 17 vials of blood work, which they took that day, and sent me home. I felt like I'd been attacked by a vampire.

The infectious disease doctor insisted I come back and meet with an internist and an endocrinologist. So, my dad once again took the day off from work and drove me three hours up and back for my appointments. Ultimately, the conclusion from the Cleveland Clinic was that they had no idea what was wrong with me or how to fix it. I was sent home, yet again, without a diagnosis and barely able to make the walk to our car.

At this point, I decided I was done with medical doctors. Considering the total lack of pay-out for my trouble, I saw no point in wasting anymore of my energy. The toll each doctor visit took on me physically and mentally was significant, as it required a lot of physical movement, social interaction, and travelling in a car—all things that were very difficult for me at that time. Clearly, I existed in a gray area that was not discussed in medical school. My case was complicated, apparently. It required someone to roll up his or her sleeves and dig and problem solve. It seemed I was not going to get that from conventional medical doctors. They had neither the time nor the appetite. What I was going to get from a conventional medical doctor was fifteen to twenty minutes, loads of expensive blood work, then a blank stare followed by, "I'm sorry, I can't help you."

It angered me. Doctors went to medical school, presumably, to help sick people. And here I was, extremely sick and in desperate need of help with not a single doctor willing to stick it out with me to figure out what was wrong. A once very active, healthy, and able-bodied young mother now found herself bedridden, virtually overnight, and living at her parents' house unable to function. I'm not a doctor, but if I was and had a patient like me walk into my office, I'd find that fact pattern completely unacceptable. I'd want to figure out what was wrong inside this person's body. If she had Lyme disease and took the requisite antibiotics, then why was she still sick? Instead of finding anyone with the desire to answer this question, I was finding doctors too pressed for time to truly help.

The medical field is a business, and I'd just learned that the hard way. Absent having a life-threatening medical emergency or illness, such as cancer, a heart attack, or broken bone, it's my opinion that you are generally better off staying away from doctors. But being angry at doctors wasn't going to help me get well, so I let it go. I came to accept that my anger was misplaced. At the end of the day, these doctors were doing their very best with what limited knowledge they had to go on. I had to stop taking it personally. Unfortunately, for as advanced as we are in modern medicine, there is still much we do not know about the human body.

I had to keep moving. What would I do next? I had no idea. For the time being, I could do nothing but stay in bed with my mom bringing me meals and praying things would start to turn around.

I stared out my bedroom window at the tree branches outside. I'd spent hour upon hour over the past few months watching from bed as the snow gave way to tiny buds that blossomed into leaves. I wondered how many more seasons I would watch come and go from that window.

CHAPTER TWO

MY STORY—PART II

"Learn to get in touch with the silence within yourself, and know that everything in life has purpose. There are no mistakes, no coincidences, all events are blessings given to us to learn from."
Elisabeth Kubler-Ross

Finding the Right Practitioners—Gound Zero

After a sobering experience at the Cleveland Clinic, and failing to believe Lyme disease was not still a factor in my poor health, I proceeded to read book after book from my bed on overcoming Lyme disease and chronic illness. I took notes on a legal pad and came up with a plan of attack. I ordered supplements and antimicrobials, and with no one but myself to guide me, I got to work.

I was my own doctor, learning on the job, so-to-speak, and while so sick I could barely keep my head up to read. It was excruciating. All I wanted to do was lay in bed, sleep and be cared for. If I wanted to get well, though, I had to figure it out. After several months of this self-care, I realized I needed a little help. The stress of always second-guessing what I was doing or what I should be doing was too much. I researched and found a very reputable LLMD in Seattle, Washington—Dr. Marty

Ross, who did Skype consultations. I immediately contacted him and set up an appointment.

Dr. Ross reviewed my medical records and concurred that I had a very clear case of chronic Lyme disease. At a minimum, he made me feel assured I was properly diagnosed. We started on a regimen of herbal medicines and pharmaceutical grade supplements, but I didn't seem to make much progress. After several months, he asked me if I would be willing to fly to Seattle so he could treat me in person. He felt I should consider going back on prescription antibiotics, but he could not prescribe anything without a face-to-face consultation. I knew that in my condition, a flight across the country was not happening. At that point, there were days where I struggled just to ride a few minutes in a car. Plus, I simply did not want to take any more antibiotics. I appreciated Dr. Ross's help and found him to be very knowledgeable, but I knew it was time to find another practitioner. I needed someone who solely focused in natural remedies.

That's when I stumbled upon a naturopath on Facebook from Montreal, Canada, who had personally recovered from Lyme disease and lupus using an entirely holistic approach. Her name was Jennifer Sierzant. The lupus part caught my attention, because I knew I also had autoimmune issues, and lupus is a serious autoimmune disease. So, once again I found myself setting up an appointment as a new patient with another practitioner.

Connecting with Jennifer was the first significant step I took to get my health under control. Over the course of many months, she laid the foundation for me to stabilize my health. Together, we worked on detoxifying my body with herbal remedies and specific foods. Then she added in gentle antimicrobials, worked with me on my diet, and taught me practical strategies for stress management. Perhaps more than anything, Jennifer affirmed my belief that natural remedies were the proper way for me to heal. Through Jennifer, I also came to learn what a true healthcare provider should do for a patient—listen, care, and dig to find the root cause of a patient's problem.

Jennifer got me on the right track, and after many months of her help, I was finding myself out of bed a little more often. I was still, for the most part, disabled, but I was certainly headed in the proper direction. I credit her for putting the brakes on my steady decline and helping me regain stability, both mentally and physically.

Moving Forward and Gaining Momentum

For seven straight years, I worked with various holistic practitioners as well as a few medical doctors who leaned into the holistic realm. By continually rotating different herbal antimicrobials, removing inflammatory foods from my diet, and working in gentle detoxifying herbs, I slowly started to improve. Over time and ever so gradually, I found myself able to do more and more things, such as grocery shop (however slowly) with my kids.

I would often compare my recovery to watching my children grow. If you are also a parent, you can probably relate to being utterly shocked to realize your children suddenly look several inches taller. You can barely believe your eyes, as you wonder how and when this happened. It was the same sort of experience measuring my health improvements. I struggled with identifying forward progress on a day-to-day basis because progress was slow and the improvements often felt trivial. But, my mom could always see it. My mother would notice what I felt were inconsequential victories—opening a jar of pickles without pain, having an improved complexion, or simply exhibiting a more cheerful disposition. Your family and friends may notice small things that you might not see, because you still feel generally awful. But keep the faith, because these small improvements are your body's way of telling you it's healing. It wasn't until I made it to the grocery store and back by myself that I acknowledged I might legitimately be getting better. But even still, I was always tempered in my assessment of progress, because at *all times* I worried about a relapse.

My next milestone came one day when I discovered a TedX talk on-line by Dr. Terry Wahls. Dr. Wahls reversed progressive multiple sclerosis using food alone. Her story was, and is, absolutely remarkable, to say the least. I soaked in every word of her lecture, and immediately bought her book—*The Wahls Protocol*. This book radically changed how I looked at food and restored my hope in a full recovery. Food became my new medicine. While I had already been improving upon my diet, I had not been as methodical and scientific about how I fueled my cells. After reading Dr. Wahls' book, I turned my focus to nutrition more so than supplementation. I still rotated antimicrobials and some specifically targeted supplements aimed at healing my gut, but my primary source of vitamins and minerals became food. This would prove to be a life-saving decision over the months and years ahead.

Over time, as I religiously stuck to Dr. Wahls' diet, many of my symptoms slowly began to fade away. Six years after initially falling sick, I no longer needed so much personal, day-to-day care, and was able to move back in with my husband where our family could live under one roof. This was also a very significant milestone in my recovery. Although I was still unable to exercise, walk more than a block slowly, or stay up for a full day without laying down several times, I was ever so gently regaining some semblance of a life.

Finally Being "Seen" at the Cleveland Clinic

In the winter of 2018, I revisited the Cleveland Clinic. This time, however, it was to the Functional Medicine Department. The Functional Medicine Department ran numerous tests, including several on my gut health. Their testing provided helpful data points with which to hone my protocol and chisel away to a state of health. I felt myself finally able to see that much talked about light at the end of the tunnel.

Also, at the Cleveland Clinic, for the first time, doctors seemed to understand my ordeal. In my first visit, after looking through my medical records and test results, the doctor looked at me and said, *"You poor thing. You've been through it, haven't you?"*

Hearing a medical professional from a prestigious medical facility say this to me almost brought me to tears. It was so strangely gratifying to be recognized. *Yes, I had been through it.* And along the way, I'd been doubted by countless doctors and others who suggested that perhaps I was just weak-minded, depressed, or exaggerating my symptoms. It was nice to finally be *seen* by a reputable doctor for what was—and is—essentially an invisible disease.

For years, I had been working 24 hours per day, 7 days per week to get well in a body that never let up on pain, fatigue, and a multitude of torturous symptoms. In a word, it was grueling. Chronic illness does not grant anyone a weekend off to regroup and gear up for the long week ahead. To the contrary, the suffering is a possible life sentence. It's difficult to muscle through each day when you're mired in a painful illness. But it's even more difficult to muscle through when you're strapped with the reality that your illness might never improve, let alone resolve. For several years, there was simply never any clarity or end in sight.

And like many who suffer from Lyme and autoimmune disease, I was always having to fake my way through life. Going out in public required me to literally put on a performance and pretend to be something I was not—a remotely healthy person. Any social gathering I attended was very painful and something to merely endure. For years, I avoided social outings almost altogether, as most days I could barely get out of bed. When I *could* get out of bed, even casual interactions felt overwhelming. And when others would see me dressed and socializing, they would just assume I was well. They could not see the hell of my daily life.

To get an idea of what this feels like, imagine for a moment you had climbed Mount Everest, but no one witnessed it. And while climbing Mount Everest, you encountered an avalanche, a blizzard, and numerous obstacles that could easily have knocked you off the mountain—or even killed you. You demonstrated an incredible work ethic and determination in conquering this mountain and tackling each unforeseen obstacle, and the sheer physicality of it took everything out of you, mentally and physically. But when you returned home, no one believed you'd climbed any mountain at all. In fact, no one thought you did much of anything. Rather, they rolled their eyes at your description of how hard your alleged feat actually was, while others suggested that enormous mountain you faced was really just a small, rolling hill. Or even more incredulous, they compared the common, everyday stresses of life to the life or death obstacles you conquered on the mountain.

Can you relate to this story? Sadly, I bet you can. *This* is what it was like for me battling Lyme and autoimmune disease, and this is what it is like for many sufferers of chronic illness.

People battling these diseases suffer on a daily basis, with the odds stacked against them to regain their health, while those around them often fail to believe or acknowledge they are even sick. There are not many other diseases like Lyme, CFS, and autoimmune disease in this regard. These invisible diseases far too frequently get dismissive, back-of-the-hand treatment from doctors, friends, and even sometimes family.

But, when all is said and done, to get well you must put the literal and figurative hurts behind you and move on. And, that is what I did.

After almost a decade of chronic and debilitating illness, it is truly miraculous to me that I have regained my current state of health. Equally miraculous is that my improvements are due almost entirely to proper and targeted nutrition.

To provide a perspective, I've listed below the symptoms to-date that I have battled. Most of them I had all at once, and then as I began to heal, they slowly started to fall away. Admittedly, I am not yet 100% healed, but I am getting there. I still have limitations with energy, but that is slowly improving each year as I adhere to the protocol set forth in the chapters ahead.

List of Symptoms:

- Debilitating fatigue (not the "I'm tired" variety)
- Systemic joint pain
- Chronic flu-like aches
- Severe Raynaud's syndrome
- Body tremors
- Painful abdominal skin rash
- Right side weakness in limbs, face, eye
- Tingling / painful hands and feet
- Yellow skin tone (particularly feet and hands)
- Bloodshot eyes
- Night sweats / fevers
- Severe insomnia
- Stabbing pains in legs
- Heavy brain fog (very difficult to carry conversations)
- Poor memory and concentration
- Light and sound sensitivity
- Feelings of water trickling down limbs and neck
- Vibrational feelings throughout body
- Heart palpitations
- Shortness of breath
- Severe post-exertion malaise
- Anxiety

Conclusion

Getting out from under this problem has been the biggest accomplishment of my life, and it's been—*by far*—the hardest I've ever worked. The self-discipline required to get well when you are totally disabled with no medical doctor to help is significant, to put it mildly. If you are to recover from a chronic illness, you must put forth an Olympic-sized effort on all fronts: mental, physical, and spiritual.

Truly to this day, I don't fully understand what exactly happened to me. Yes, I was diagnosed with Lyme disease one full year after the on-set of symptoms. But was that my initial problem? I don't know. And as time went on, I quit testing positive for Lyme disease, but was still fully sick. I initially had very high autoimmune markers, but they simmered down as my health improved. Perhaps the antibiotic I took set off a cascade of autoimmunity in my body, which wore down my immune system and enabled a dormant Lyme infection to come to life? No medical professional has ever been able to tell me with total certainty precisely what went wrong.

Sometimes, the bottom line is that you are simply sick. What you "have" may not ever be fully fleshed out. But that does not mean you cannot get yourself back to a state of health. A sick and out of balance body needs to find homeostasis. It needs you to take away toxic burdens and replenish it with a nutrient-dense diet that fuels deep healing. It also needs you to be gentle and give yourself time to heal. That means reducing your stress load, getting plenty of sleep, and caring for yourself just like you would a best friend—all things we will discuss in the chapters ahead!

CHAPTER THREE

UNDERSTANDING MYSTERY ILLNESSES— Lyme Disease, Chronic Fatigue Syndrome ("CFS"), Fibromyalgia & Autoimmune Disease

"Hard times don't create heroes. It is during the hard times when the 'hero' within us is revealed."
Bob Riley

My experience with "mystery illness" involved Lyme disease, chronic fatigue syndrome ("CFS"), fibromyalgia, and autoimmune illness. These illnesses can be difficult to diagnose and treat, and often patients are told they have one illness when really it's another. It's very easy to fall into a black void of illness, not ever knowing exactly what is wrong. Symptoms overlap, testing is murky, and doctors are at a loss as to how to treat you.

Let's take a look at each of these mystery illnesses individually.

1. LYME DISEASE & TICK-BORNE ILLNESS

Lyme disease and tick-borne illnesses derail the lives of hundreds of thousands of people annually, both in the US and around the globe.[6] Lyme disease is a bacterial infection typically transferred by a black legged tick.[7] Other tick-borne illnesses may accompany a Lyme infection, such as babesia, bartonella, ehrlichiosis, tularemia, or Rocky Mountain spotted fever, to name a few. These co-infections, as they are often called, may be transferred by various ticks, such as the lone star tick, Rocky Mountain wood tick, brown dog tick, American dog tick, Gulf Coast tick, or Pacific Coast tick, among others.[8] Ticks may also carry viruses, such as Powassan virus, which has a ten percent fatality rate.[9]

Truthfully, Lyme disease and its co-infections are much more than a simple infection. More precisely, Lyme disease is an infection-induced systemic breakdown inside the body that, when left improperly treated, opens the floodgates for all sorts of other problems to take hold, such as autoimmune diseases, parasitic infections, adrenal fatigue, and food sensitivities. Symptoms can include severe joint pain, crippling fatigue, insomnia, skin rashes, body tremors, cognition and memory problems, paralysis, Bell's Palsy, night sweats, chronic flu-like aches, and more. Such symptoms can be endless and unrelenting. Reflecting back now on my experience, I actually feel a little short-changed telling people I simply contracted an infection. Many do not realize that Lyme disease can become a very complicated and debilitating illness, compromising numerous body systems at once.

Incredulously, Lyme disease sufferers may appear perfectly normal and healthy on the outside, but all the while they are dying on the inside. Lyme is often an invisible disease that causes many to suffer alone. Family and friends can fail to appreciate the degree of pain and suffering because nothing looks outwardly amiss. I used to hate it when, while feeling very ill, someone would tell me how wonderful I looked. Looking great while so seriously sick isn't much comfort and actually works against you in many ways. Friends and loved ones may completely dismiss your struggle and fail to provide the help and compassion you desperately need. Even your family doctor may dismiss you as depressed, or worse, as a hypochondriac because your tests are "normal" and you do not appear sick. At my sickest, I truly felt as though I needed a prop, such as a cast or wheelchair, to properly convey to the outside world how I felt.

Difficulty with Diagnosis and Treatment

Almost worse than the disease itself is the archaic diagnosis process and subsequent treatment, or lack thereof. Sadly, many people who suffer from this disease do not even know they've contracted it, as according to the CDC, testing is about as accurate as a coin toss. The standard Lyme disease antibody test governed by the CDC and given by medical professionals may be wrong about half of the time or more.[10] The problem with this test is that it looks for antibodies to the infection rather than the infection itself. In the early stages of a Lyme disease infection, the sufferer may not have produced the requisite antibodies to test positive, or the immune system simply may not have launched the proper response. For this reason, the CDC reported in 2014 that the number of Lyme disease cases in the US has been largely under reported.[11] Of course this means that, regardless of how well-intentioned your doctor is, your odds of being properly diagnosed and treated are sub-optimal. You could very easily walk out of a doctor's office fully sick with Lyme disease and yet be told you are perfectly well. Or, you may be told you have chronic fatigue syndrome, or fibromyalgia, or even multiple sclerosis. There are numerous documented cases of people diagnosed with MS who treated for Lyme disease instead and put their "MS" into remission.[12]

Unfortunately, once you test negative for Lyme disease on the antiquated test currently offered, your doctor will more than likely refuse to further consider a Lyme infection. You may have had the tell-tale bullseye rash, as I did, and along with that rash every symptom of Lyme disease, but without the positive test result, you will risk being viewed as a hypochondriac if you push the issue. While the nation's top Lyme Literate Medical Doctors (LLMDs) attest that Lyme disease requires a clinical diagnosis and not one based solely on blood test results, the medical community at large relies completely on test results.

Further, most traditional medical doctors refuse to acknowledge that Lyme disease can become chronic. Many sufferers continue to have debilitating symptoms after being treated with the requisite amount of antibiotics recommended by the CDC. If this happens to you, you are on your own. You will likely be told, as I was, that you have developed chronic fatigue syndrome, fibromyalgia, or some other syndrome. It is important to keep in mind, as my LLMD very astutely put it to me, that CFS and fibromyalgia are nothing more than a set of symptoms with an unknown cause. These diagnoses, if you can even call them that, serve no useful purpose to the patient. They are your doctor's way of saying, "I have no idea what is wrong with you." But, more on that later.

After labeling you with a meaningless diagnosis, almost invariably the doctor adds further injury by encouraging you to add prescription drugs such as Cymbalta or other anti-depressants, steroids, and/or pain medications to mask symptoms. Meanwhile, neither the doctor nor the patient has any idea what is actually wrong inside the body.

Conversely, any LLMD, functional medicine doctor, or naturopath experienced in Lyme disease will contend that a patient who continues to exhibit symptoms after initial treatment, regardless of any subsequent negative test results, has an unresolved chronic infection that likely still requires treatment.

This is where the politics of Lyme disease arise. Treating a Lyme disease patient with antibiotics for a longer duration than recommended by the CDC puts a medical doctor at risk of losing his or her medical license.

Compounding the problem is the unreliable testing previously discussed. If there isn't a blood test showing a patient is still positive for Lyme, there is little for a medical doctor to hang his or her hat on, so-to-speak, in order to prescribe long-term antibiotics. It is quite understandable that very few medical doctors are willing to stick their necks out for chronic Lyme disease patients. And hence, the reason LLMDs are so difficult to find. Fortunately, alternative medical professionals are not bound by such restrictions because they do not deal exclusively in prescription drugs, but rather in natural antimicrobial and over-the-counter herbal protocols.

Even if you *are* treated by a competent LLMD who fully understands this disease, you may still find your head spinning from the aggressive treatment plan that is recommended. A standard approach to a chronic Lyme infection by many LLMDs is to flood the body with oral or intravenous antibiotics. Never mind that Lyme disease may have taken up residence in your body due to a weakened immune system or gut permeability—conditions that could be greatly exacerbated by an aggressive antibiotic regimen. Antibiotics are foreign and toxic by nature to the body, particularly when taken for the duration and dose required to kill a chronic Lyme disease infection, and they are quite taxing on an already stressed system. For some, they are absolutely *the* answer, particularly in early stages. But, for many with late-stage and chronic disease, they are not. With a chronic Lyme disease infection, you may need to be open to various treatment options, including natural and holistic ones, which may take more time to work but are gentler on the body.

The Cost of Lyme Disease

The physical toll of Lyme disease is matched only by its monetary toll. Most LLMDs do not accept health insurance and may charge anywhere from $300 to well over $1200 per visit. Now, consider it takes months to several years to clear a chronic Lyme disease infection and do the math.

LLMDs are also sparsely scattered throughout the country, requiring many ill patients to travel long distances for appointments, thereby racking up significant travel and lodging costs.

Testing is also typically not covered by insurance and is expensive. Because Lyme disease seldom comes by itself, you will need to be tested for a slew of other infections, all likely out of pocket. Medications are also typically not covered by insurance, especially if you were not positive for Lyme disease via CDC testing guidelines, and many are not. Insurance companies often do not recognize your disease if it was not diagnosed using the CDC's western blot test, which, as stated earlier, is wrong half of the time. In this event, patients may find themselves spending thousands of dollars per month just for antibiotics and dietary supplements needed to properly battle the disease.

If you think medicine and doctor appointments will be your only expense, think again. You will likely need to drastically overhaul your diet, requiring you to spend money on more expensive items at the grocery store, such as organic vegetables and grass-fed organic meats. Dietary supplements to replenish a burned out and taxed body will be absolutely critical. These supplements can cost hundreds of dollars per month.

And what happens to your career during all of this? You can pretty much forget about working during treatment. Your career plans will be on hold indefinitely, which means you will be spending significantly more while earning significantly less. Being approved for disability insurance is difficult, as Lyme disease not diagnosed via CDC testing may not be recognized as a condition by the Disability Office. Further, even if you are approved, the process can take several years to complete. Getting well can easily cause a person to go bankrupt.

This leads to the final casualty of Lyme disease: your personal life. Many chronically ill patients find themselves isolated and alone, no longer able to care for their families, socialize, or participate in life as they once did. Over time, friends and family disappear from your life as you spend most of your days in bed unable to function. If you are fortunate like me, you have family that will help you, but many are not. It can be very difficult to find someone with the patience to help a chronically sick person, as being a caregiver is intensely stressful and time consuming. Often a person's only available caregiver is his or her spouse, and this can quickly erode a marriage.

2. CHRONIC FATIGUE SYNDROME ("CFS") & FIBROMYALGIA

Chronic fatigue syndrome and fibromyalgia are two insidious diseases that quietly decimate the lives of millions of people each year. According to the CDC, one-million or more Americans currently suffer from CFS and approximately four million suffer from fibromyalgia.[13] Neither illness has a known cause or a known cure.

For purposes of this book, I group CFS with fibromyalgia because the two are very closely related. With CFS, the main complaint is overwhelming exhaustion that is not relieved by rest. With CFS you likely also experience body pain, but it is secondary to fatigue. With fibromyalgia, the situation is reversed. Body pain is the primary complaint and any associated fatigue is secondary. Both diseases cause a myriad of symptoms ranging from joint pain, fatigue, depression, and anxiety to insomnia, memory and cognitive problems, muscle twitching, headaches and migraines, etc.[14]

A patient may get an alternating diagnosis of fibromyalgia or CFS because symptoms wax and wane—as was my case. You may have started out with a fibromyalgia diagnosis and watched that morph into CFS, as debilitating fatigue became your primary problem. While a medical doctor may distinguish between the two illnesses, both CFS and fibromyalgia essentially equate to a set of mysterious symptoms without a known cause. Either diagnosis is completely meaningless. Imagine going to your doctor with a headache and fatigue and you get diagnosed with "Headache & Fatigue Syndrome," or "HFS." It's *that* ridiculous. Your doctor will likely tell you that, while it is not curable, it may be "managed" by prescription anti-depressants, pain medications, and sleeping pills. If you have a really progressive doctor, he or she may also recommend light stretching, yoga and meditation to help with pain and sleep. And that is likely as far as you will get.

The real-life implications of CFS and fibromyalgia are devastating, and identical to what I've previously discussed with Lyme disease. You cannot function, and meanwhile you look perfectly healthy. You can no longer work, but have difficulty getting approved for disability due to very poor diagnostic testing. Often times, people are diagnosed with CFS or fibromyalgia only to later find they really have Lyme disease. Symptoms overlap and doctors rely on blood tests that are not always reliable.

The emotional and physical toll of being sick and unable to figure out what you really "have" or what is really going wrong is completely deflating. People get depressed because of their seemingly hopeless situation, and rightfully so.

3. AUTOIMMUNE DISEASE

Approximately 20% of the US population suffers from an autoimmune disease, 78% of whom are women.[15] Some of the more common autoimmune diseases include lupus, rheumatoid arthritis ("RA"), Crohn's disease, Hashimoto's thyroiditis, psoriasis, and multiple sclerosis ("MS").

Autoimmunity occurs when the body's immune system mistakenly attacks itself. A healthy immune system, when faced with a pathogen, will create antibodies with which to launch an attack against the "foreign" invader. These antibodies essentially kill the pathogen, and the person then returns to health. With autoimmunity, the person suffers a dysfunctional or overactive immune system, and the body incorrectly identifies its own tissue as a foreign invader. So, you create antibodies literally against yourself. This creates a wide litany of symptoms. The autoimmune disease you are ultimately diagnosed with depends upon what part of the body is attacked.[16]

For example, with lupus, the body can attack various tissues, often times the skin, kidneys, heart or nervous system. Rheumatoid arthritis ("RA") affects the soft tissue of the joints, causing severe joint pain and damage. With Crohn's disease, the immune system attacks the cells of the digestive tract. In the case of Hashimoto's thyroiditis, the thyroid gland is attacked. With psoriasis, the skin is attacked, and with multiple sclerosis, the central nervous system is attacked.[17]

All of these diseases have the same underlying problem: the immune system is misfiring and there is no known cause or cure. The symptoms are very similar to those discussed with Lyme disease, CFS, and fibromyalgia in that they are wide ranging. Sufferers may experience joint pain, rashes, muscle weakness, body aches, fatigue, cognition and memory problems, body tremors, gastrointestinal issues, paralysis, and vision impairment, etc.[18] Treatments are aimed at reducing immune system activity, which inevitably has the effect of increasing one's susceptibility to other infections and disease. Such treatments are never curative and only prolong a guaranteed decline.

Conclusion

We are so advanced in many ways when it comes to healthcare, and yet there is still so much doctors have to learn about the human body. I simply never contemplated the possibility that I could become disabled with an illness that no doctor could properly diagnose or treat, until it happened. Sadly, I am not alone. What happened to me happens to millions of people every year. These "mystery illnesses" desperately need more funding and study, as current treatment options fall far too short.

So, what do you do if you find yourself sick with one of these illnesses? It certainly seems a grim picture—if you accept current and often ineffective medical treatments. I urge you not to do that. No matter where you find yourself now, improvement and even a complete reversal of your symptoms may be possible. Take action this very moment and remain patient, committed, and disciplined. This book will equip you with the tools you need to begin your journey back to health.

CHAPTER FOUR

COMING TO TERMS

"We may encounter many defeats, but we must not be defeated."
Maya Angelou

As the saying goes, your health is your wealth. Sadly, few of us appreciate our health until it is gone. And once it's gone, it is very hard to get back. But it's not impossible. In fact, it is probably more possible than most people would even begin to believe. Before we dig in, though, there are three basic truths about chronic illness that you will need to reconcile.

First, YOU are Responsible for Your Health

We are all personally responsible for our own health. Growing up, I had always been lead to believe that doctors kept us all well, and that's somewhat accurate. But the truth is, doctors are not wizards. *You* are the one living inside your body making each and every day-to-day decision. Every single thing you do to your body on a daily basis, from applying moisturizer to enjoying pizza and beer with friends on the weekend, has an impact over time. There are no mulligans when it comes to your health—all of it matters. Suffice it to say, to get well, you must take ownership of your current state of health.

When considering healthcare, people generally fail to recognize their own personal power. We place so much power in the hands of our doctors and so very little power in our own hands. Let me assure you, there is much we can do on our own through proper nutrition and lifestyle to reverse illness. Yet, most people scoff at the very idea of food reversing disease. I've been called a quack more times than not for my personal take on nutrition and health. Too many people have simply been brainwashed to believe they must take a pharmaceutical drug to get well, and if none exists, that they are sentenced to a life of agony.

I was once one of "those" people. When I fell sick in January of 2012, I felt helpless absent a doctor telling me what to do. When doctors essentially washed their hands of me, I felt like I'd been abandoned on a deserted island with nothing but my own bare hands to get me home. I was terrified and felt powerless. I had absolutely no inkling that the food I ate could be contributing to my problems, nor that my problems had likely manifested when I was a child eating Captain Crunch cereal for breakfast, Wonder Bread sandwiches for lunch, and pasta filled casseroles for dinner. Nor did it occur to me as an adult, when I was exercising regularly and eating a "healthy" low-fat diet of deli-meat sandwiches, milk, yogurt, breakfast cereals, pasta, and the occasional salad with a vegetable or fruit thrown in for good measure, that I was contributing in any way to a disease state.

Does this sound familiar? Do you generally eat "well" and exercise, but still find yourself sick? If it does, you're not alone.

Most people have no idea what it truly means to eat well and properly care for their body. Throwing some fruits and vegetables into your diet each day and squeezing in a workout does *not* mean you're taking care of yourself properly. Rest assured, we will get into this much more deeply in the chapters ahead. But know this: your daily routine, which encompasses everything from sleep, stress management, toxin exposure, exercise, and diet all conspire to determine your current state of health.

This means that your health largely depends upon your personal daily choices. So from here on out, make them good ones.

Second, There are NO Magic Pills to Regain Your Health

Chronic illnesses, such as Lyme disease, CFS, MS, or fibromyalgia are the end-result of many different things going wrong over a long period of time.[19] In other words, when you eventually fall sick, it's a complicated mess running amok inside your body. And suffice it to say, there are rarely any simple answers or miracle cures. In fact, many (if not all) of the drugs your doctor may offer for these illnesses will simply mask symptoms. At best, they may make you feel more comfortable as your condition continues to decline. At worst, they may make you more sick.

I'm not suggesting that you should never take prescription medication. Prescription drugs definitely have their place. Modern medicine is a wonderful thing, and we are all fortunate to live in this day in age where doctors have so many tools at their disposal. If you have suffered through anything acute such as pneumonia, cancer, or even a broken leg, certainly you are grateful for antibiotics, chemotherapy, and pain medication.

But the fact remains that *all* drugs come with side-effects, and as a society, we are often using pharmaceutical drugs unnecessarily. To demonstrate this point, consider that from 1997 to 2016, the total number of prescriptions filled by Americans increased by 85%, while at the same time, the US population only increased by 21 percent.[20] Without a doubt, we are too quick to overlook and underestimate the body's innate ability to heal itself when given the proper environment—a sound diet, proper sleep, and exercise.

Third, It's Possible to Get Well Without a Diagnosis

Healing is possible, even if your search for a diagnosis goes unanswered, by following basic principles in functional medicine and taking a broad approach to your health. Functional and holistic medicine view the body as a whole and consider disease the end-result of a handful of core foundational problems.

According to Dr. Bill Rahl's, who cured himself of chronic Lyme disease using herbal remedies and functional medicine principles, there are seven main causes of disease. They are as follows:[21]

1. Nutritional stress
2. Emotional stress
3. Toxins
4. Physical stress
5. Free radicals / inflammation
6. Radiation
7. Microbes

By properly addressing the areas outlined above by Dr. Rahls, and following the protocol set forth in the coming chapters, your body will begin shifting toward health, regardless of your current diagnosis—or lack thereof.

To better understand how one treatment plan can help reverse many different illnesses, you must understand that identical root problem(s) in ten different people may manifest in ten different sets of symptoms or illnesses.[22] For instance, the person whose immune system allowed MS to take root may have the same core problem(s) as the person whose immune system allowed CFS or Lyme disease to spread like wild fire throughout the body. To demonstrate, my health crisis involved Lyme disease, CFS, and autoimmune illness. But, I personally know people who put cancer into remission using the same principles I outline in the coming chapters.

Simply stated, in many instances, disease is disease, and it doesn't much matter what you are calling it.

As Dr. Terry Wahls, the brilliant doctor and author of *The Wahls Protocol*, wrote when discussing autoimmune disease:

> Whether you are diagnosed with multiple sclerosis or rheumatoid arthritis or systemic lupus or inflammatory bowel disease—or whether you are told your symptoms are "idiopathic" (meaning we don't know what is causing them)—depends largely on how your disease looks on the outside. Inside, the distinction between these autoimmune diseases is, frankly, fairly arbitrary, although there are different ways to view, think about, and understand what is happening when cellular dysfunction gains a foothold…[h]owever, the fact remains that inside the body, health problems begin in the cells.[23]

If your experience is anything like mine, you've already been to a gazillion doctors. And they have almost all failed you. Maybe you have a diagnosis at this point, maybe you don't. Or, you have a diagnosis but are not sure if it is reliable. All you know is that you feel terrible every day you wake up, and you can't figure out how to get well.

Over the course of many years, I was diagnosed with different things at different times. Initially, I was diagnosed with Lyme disease, but at some point along the way, I quit testing positive for active Lyme infection. My inflammation markers also went down, and yet, I still had debilitating symptoms. I was told I had developed CFS, then fibromyalgia, and then a post-Lyme-disease-syndrome that had no cure. Other illnesses, such as MS, were mentioned, but I had simply tired of testing. I couldn't do it anymore.

I found myself at a crossroads. Should I continue down this path in search of another diagnosis with medical doctors whose only recourse would be a pharmaceutical drug? Or, did I want to find another way to truly heal my body?

I decided I was going to stop looking to doctors, invasive testing, and external sources for answers. The medical profession had done nothing for me up to that point, except wear me out mentally, physically, and financially. This decision was truly gratifying, because I was so tired of being on the hamster wheel of perpetually chasing down a diagnosis, upset because I couldn't confidently put a name to my symptoms.

Don't get me wrong, it would have been nice to know exactly what was going on inside my body. And if you are able to achieve a clear and concise diagnosis, you are fortunate. A precise diagnosis gives you something to confidently direct your efforts towards so you can implement a targeted treatment. It also makes it easier for friends and family to understand why you are in bed all day. When you can no longer participate in life, people want to know why. A simple answer such as, "she's got Lyme disease," is much easier than going over a litany of mysterious symptoms.

But for some people, a clear and accurate diagnosis may not be attainable. Your problem may not yet be well understood by doctors, and testing for many chronic conditions is often unreliable. Invasive testing and never-ending doctor visits take their toll on a sick body. Eventually, you have to weigh the benefit of these visits with the burden they create. For me, letting go of this need to know was very cathartic. Over time, I also realized that putting a name to my symptoms really was more for *other* people, and not so much for me or my health. At the end of the day, I considered myself to be one thing—sick.

So, exhausted, but finally believing in functional and holistic medicine and the power of nutrition, I redirected my focus from wondering what I "had" to instead determining what my body needed to support it in healing. It became my belief that no matter my ailment, if I properly supported my body, it would do what it was designed to do—fix itself.

If you've been to endless doctors at this point and are still uncertain of what you "have," do not lose hope. By all means, continue going for testing if a diagnosis seems attainable. I'm certainly not encouraging anyone to be derelict in his or her search for answers. It's also very important to rule out potentially serious illnesses, such as cancer or genetic disorders, and to monitor conditions such as thyroid disease. But take comfort that healing is certainly possible absent a specific diagnosis.

Conclusion

So, to sum up:

(1) **YOU—and only YOU—are responsible for your health and the decisions you make each day relative to your body;**

(2) **There are NO magic pills to get you well; and**

(3) **Healing is possible—even without a diagnosis—by following the principles outlined in this book and basic tenets of functional medicine.**

These points may take time to digest, but they are basic truths upon which your healing will begin.

PART II

The Heavy Lifting of Getting Well

CHAPTER FIVE

A CRASH COURSE IN GUT HEALTH & YOUR ROADMAP TO HEALTH

"It is always the simple that produces the marvelous."
Amelia Bar

In the following chapters, I present an eight-step recovery plan to reclaim your health, revealing modalities that are not widely known, but that worked incredibly well for me. Before we begin, however, I must underscore the importance of gut health, as sound gut health will be the foundation to your healing. Understanding the basics of gut health will be absolutely critical to your success, and it must be addressed before we officially begin.

Why Your Gut Matters

As Hippocrates very astutely said, "All disease begins in the gut." If I could tell you only one thing to restore your health, it would be this: heal your gut. If you are sick with anything, be it chronic Lyme disease, MS, arthritis, chronic headaches, psoriasis, or certainly any major disease or autoimmune illness, your gut is in rough shape and you may suffer from leaky gut syndrome.

Leaky Gut Syndrome

Leaky gut syndrome occurs when the tight junctions inside the walls of your intestine become loose or permeable.[24] When these junctions become loose, whatever passes through the walls of the small intestine may leak into your bloodstream.[25]

Naturopathic doctors and holistic practitioners often assert that autoimmunity results from leaky gut syndrome, as particles that should have passed fully enclosed in the intestine instead enter the bloodstream causing the body's immune system to go haywire and launch an attack upon itself.[26] Functional medicine practitioners also largely believe leaky gut syndrome is likely to exist in any patient suffering a chronic illness, particularly serious and debilitating illnesses such as chronic Lyme disease, MS, or CFS. I can personally attest, with absolute certainty, that once I honed in on leaky gut syndrome, my symptoms significantly began to improve.

What exactly causes a leaky gut is not known, but some practitioners suspect it is due to a poor diet, stress, and toxins. One theory is that a hormone called zonulin, which regulates the gut's permeability, becomes activated by the aforementioned stressors and a leaky gut ensues.[27]

According to Ronald Grisanti D.C., D.A.B.C.O., D.A.C.B.N., M.S. of Functional Medicine University (FMU):

> Leaky Gut Syndrome (LGS) is a major cause of disease and dysfunction in modern society, and accounts for at least 50% of chronic complaints, as confirmed by laboratory tests. In LGS, the epithelium on the villi of the small intestine becomes inflamed and irritated, which allows metabolic and microbial toxins of the small intestines to flood into the blood stream. This event compromises the liver, the lymphatic system,

and the immune response including the endocrine system. Some of the most incurable diseases are caused by this exact mechanism, where the body attacks its own tissues. This is commonly called autoimmune disease. It is often the primary cause of the following common conditions: asthma, food allergies, chronic sinusitis, eczema, urticaria, migraine, irritable bowel, fungal disorders, fibromyalgia, and inflammatory joint disorders, including rheumatoid arthritis. It also contributes to PMS, uterine fibroid, and breast fibroid. Leaky Gut Syndrome is often the real basis for chronic fatigue syndrome and pediatric immune deficiencies.[28]

Please know, traditional medical doctors will not likely diagnose you with leaky gut syndrome. There is yet to be direct proof of its existence in most diseases, but it has absolutely been shown to exist in Crohn's disease, celiac disease, in individuals receiving chemotherapy, and in those who excessively use alcohol or aspirin.[29] Several studies have also shown increased intestinal permeability in relatives of people with Crohn's disease who are at an increased risk of later developing the illness.[30]

So, while the medical community may be at odds over leaky gut syndrome, no one disputes that gut health is fundamental to our overall health.[31] In fact, an enormous part of our immune system operates from our intestines, where certain cells on the gut lining create very large quantities of antibodies.[32] Quite interestingly, in a recent study, the role of gut health on the immune system was highlighted after mice afflicted with an experimental form of MS recovered by manipulating their guts' microbiomes.[33] Scientists have also discovered that our gut produces about 90% of our body's serotonin, a critical hormone for mood and feelings of well-being.[34] In other words, even health conditions such as depression, which most people consider a condition of the brain, are actually largely a condition of the gut!

Below is an excerpt from the NYU Langone Health Division of Gastroenterology, Department of Medicine's web site, addressing the critical role our gut plays in our well-being:

> According to Dr. Lisa Ganjhu, clinical assistant professor of medicine at NYU Langone Medical Center, the gastrointestinal system is more than the body's primary site of taking in and absorbing nutrients. This system of critical digestive organs also acts as a type of switchboard or communication center to and from the brain, and functions as one of the body's frontlines in the fight against disease. "*Our gut plays a major role, not only in our gastrointestinal health, but in the health and well-being of the entire body,*" Dr. Ganjhu said. "*All foods we eat are in communication with immune receptors in the digestive tract, triggering hormones and various cell types that help the body with its immune function,*" Dr. Ganjhu explained.[35]

In short, your gut is central to every function in your body, and if you fail to improve your gut health, you may never get well.

Fortunately, as you implement each of the eight steps outlined in my plan, you can restore your gut health. And with improved gut health, I predict you will reduce or even reverse many of the chronic symptoms from which you currently suffer.

Now that you understand why gut health is so vitally important, let's take a look at my eight-step recovery plan in more detail.

Eight-Step Recovery Plan

1. Implement a Targeted & Nutrient-Dense Diet
2. Balance Your Hormones
3. Combat Infection with Targeted Herbal Protocols
4. Restore Proper Balance to Your Microbiome
5. Implement Gentle Detox & Support Modalities
6. Restore Energy with Targeted Nutrition, Exercise, and Supplementation
7. Detoxify Your Environment
8. Implement Effective Coping & Stress Management Strategies

The plan I've set forth in the pages ahead is the plan I *wish* I had when I fell sick in January 2012. Unfortunately for me, doctors were of no help, and I had nowhere to turn for answers. I was left on my own to figure it out. While acutely ill and scared for my future, I spent countless hours performing extensive and pain-staking research—scouring books, listening to webinars, and meeting with endless medical practitioners, from traditional western medicine to holistic and Chinese medicine. The culmination of my efforts is succinctly summed up for you in the chapters ahead. I did a tremendous amount of legwork, so you don't have to. Instead, you can devote all of your time and energy to actual healing.

It's time for your healing journey to begin! Let's turn the page and get to work.

CHAPTER SIX

RECOVERY STEP #1—Implement a Targeted & Nutrient-Dense Diet

"The doctor of the future will no longer treat the human frame with drugs, but rather will cure and prevent disease with nutrition."
Thomas Edison

A targeted and nutrient-dense diet is the most critical component to health and healing. There are numerous healing diets to consider, however, most are fundamentally similar. A healing diet should exclude dairy, added sugar, and gluten, while including a nutrient-dense variety of leafy greens, low starch vegetables, healthy fats, and colorful low-sugar fruits and berries. Protein sources should be grass-fed, hormone and antibiotic free, and humanely raised. If this sounds impossible, don't panic. It takes time to master, but you can do it. Just don't make every change all at once.

Feeding Your Cells To Heal—What to Eat and What to Avoid

The diet I follow is presented in the book, *The Wahls Protocol*, by Dr. Terry Wahls. Her diet has truly been the cornerstone to my healing, although I have tweaked it along the way for various reasons, which I will discuss later. In her book, Dr. Wahls outlines a very specific approach to eating greens, vegetables, fruits, lean meats and seafood (among other things), and you can easily determine how much of each you need based on her recommendations.[36] She goes to great lengths explaining how, why, and what foods are damaging to your cells and likely preventing you from getting well. I've read countless books on nutrition since falling sick, and in my estimation, Dr. Wahls is THE authority on nutrition. Consider her book mandatory reading for the weekend!

In the pages ahead, I will review some basic guidelines to follow when developing your own personal diet, but Dr. Wahls should be your Bible and your authority on all matters relating to food. A main premise of Dr. Wahls' diet, and any healing diet, is that you must avoid foods to which you are sensitive and those which contain gluten, dairy, and added sugars (and by definition anything processed), all of which are immune system disruptors.[37]

So, what should you eat and what should you avoid? Let's take a look.

Elimination Diet & Food Sensitivity Testing

Because everyone is different with a unique biology, there truly is no one-size-fits-all diet that outlines precisely what you should eat. So, you are going to have to do your own digging and determine which foods are working for you and which are working against you. While spinach, for example, is widely accepted as a "superfood," for some people, it may create an autoimmune response. You will need to be a literal detective relative to your food intake, taking notice as to how you feel after you eat specific foods. This is often referred to as an "elimination diet," meaning you remove all the food items from your diet that you believe to be inflammatory, and then over time slowly add them back in. Each time you add an item back in, you go slowly and wait to see if you have any sort of negative response.

If you need to, start a food diary so you can take note of any reactions you have to particular foods. The one thing that must remain constant, regardless of any sensitivities or reactions, is that your food sources need to be "clean," meaning as free of pesticides, antibiotics, heavy metals (in the case of seafood), and other toxins as possible. Generally speaking, if it doesn't come from the earth or the ocean and isn't organic, don't eat it. Ingredients in any recipe or meal should be very simple. If you can't pronounce it, you probably should not eat it. Read labels, or better yet, avoid foods with labels as they are more likely to be processed.

You can also order a food sensitivity blood test over the internet, or ask your practitioner to administer one. These tests are relatively inexpensive and allow you to gauge your body's immune response to hundreds of foods. Keep in mind, this is not a food allergy test, but merely a test for sensitivities to certain foods. It is also not an exact science. Life Extension is a company that sells an affordable test that I found useful, but there are many others. If you're like me and have a hard time with the elimination diet (because my body was so out of whack, a reaction was hard to decipher), then this may be a good route to take. Most practitioners recommend the elimination diet over these blood tests, as these tests can be unreliable. My experience with food sensitivity testing was positive, though, and I did one or two each year for several years. I found that as my symptoms decreased, my sensitivity tests reflected it. Each time I tested, there would be fewer and fewer foods to which I reacted.

FOODS TO AVOID

1. Gluten

Grains such as wheat, barley, rye, and oats contain gluten and should be eliminated. Gluten is a protein made of two components, gliadins and glutenins. Neither component is easily broken down during digestion.[38] And when they enter into the bloodstream, some people create antibodies and hence an autoimmune reaction.[39] This leads to inflammation, which then leads to disease.[40] Grains in general are also broken down into sugar by our bodies. Too much sugar feeds the bad bugs in our guts, which in turn tips the scales of health against us. When the bad bugs outnumber the good bugs, illness ensues. I highly recommend slowly but surely removing starchy grains, such as white potatoes and bread, completely out of your diet. At a minimum, remove anything containing gluten and limit other grains to one or two servings per week.

2. Dairy

Dairy is also often a trigger for many people. It contains a form of protein called casein that may be very difficult for the body to digest. Casein consumption has also been linked to cancer.[41] When you are sick, the last thing you want to do is put an unnecessary strain on the body. Cheese and milk are not worth a lifetime of illness, so get rid of them.

3. Added Sugar and Processed Food

Sugar and processed foods need little explanation. At this point, we all know that added sugar is absolutely terrible for your body. Ensure your sugar intake is only from low-sugar fruits and vegetables. Also remember, sugar is sugar. Whether you're eating 100 grams of sugar from fruit or 100 grams of sugar from ice cream, your body does not know the difference. Be keenly aware of your sugar intake, and avoid any foods—"healthy" or not—that contain high amounts of sugar. As for processed foods, they contain all sorts of toxic additives, ranging from unhealthy fats, to toxic dyes, and preservatives. If you must eat processed foods, ensure they are as minimally processed as possible.

4. Anything You Are Sensitive To

As discussed previously, no matter what the food is, whether it be kale or a blueberry, if it creates a symptom in you, avoid it. Implement the elimination diet and pay close attention to those foods that make your immune system fire up.

FOODS TO ENJOY

1. Leafy Greens, Colorful Vegetables, and Low-Sugar Fruit

Eat from the rainbow. You want most of your daily calories to be from dark, leafy greens and colorful fruits and vegetables. I rotate various greens every week to ensure I am getting all sorts of nutrients from as many sources as possible. In other words, don't just eat spinach and kale every day. You want to mix it up and eat a wide variety of greens. You also want to ensure you are eating sulfur vegetables, such cauliflower, broccoli, and brussel sprouts—basically anything that smells.

When it comes to fruits and vegetables, you want to ensure what you are eating is not just colorful on the outside, but the entire way through. You also want to opt for low-sugar fruits. For example, blueberries would be a better option than an apple or banana. Both apples and bananas are higher in sugar than blueberries and will likely be less nutrient-dense as noted by the lack of color beneath the skin.

2. High Quality Meat in Moderation

I believe, based on Dr. Wahls' recommendations, that you must also eat animal protein. This is a somewhat controversial position, as many people are vegan and have legitimate reasons for not eating animal protein. To heal, however, your cells need the amino acids, Co-Q10, fatty acids, and other nutrients found in animal protein.[42] This does not mean you've got a green light to eat enormous amounts of animal protein. To the contrary, protein is limited on *The Wahls Protocol*. But, if you adhere to *The Wahls Protocol*, you will need to work red meat and fish into your diet.[43]

I will also caution that this does not mean eating processed deli meat (ever) or ground beef every night. You will want to limit your red meat to grass fed, humanely-raised, and nutrient-dense meat. Organ meat is an ideal choice, as it is nutrient-dense and an excellent source of iron, vitamin A, B vitamins, and Co-Q10. An easy and palatable way to work organ meat into your diet is to order beef liverwurst from US Wellness Meats. This farm ensures all of its meat is from high quality, grass fed sources. US Wellness Meat's beef liverwurst has liver, heart, and kidney meat—outstanding for your cellular health. They also sell a wonderful variety of other quality meats, including salmon. Fish is necessary for the obvious reason that it supplies the body with omega-3 fatty acids, essential for your brain and critical for fighting inflammation. Always ensure your fish is wild-caught and not farm-raised. Fish in "the wild," i.e., their natural habitat, eat a healthy and normal diet, whereas farm-raised fish are often malnourished and raised in cramped and unnatural living environments. Yes, you could simply supplement with fish oil for fatty acids, but fish and seafood are loaded with other nutrients and are the best source of what your body needs. Any time you can get your nutrients from food instead of a pill, do it.

3. Bone Broth & Hydrolyzed Collagen

Bone broth and hydrolyzed collagen are main staples in my diet for improving gut health. Because bone broth and collagen contain the amino acid L-glutamine, both are thought to be particularly helpful in healing leaky gut syndrome.

The gut is lined with cells called enterocytes which regenerate every 2-3 weeks. These enterocytes prefer L-glutamine for fuel. So, L-glutamine provides these cells the energy they need to heal.[44] While L-glutamine is found naturally in bone broth, it's also found in other foods, such as meat, fish, and spinach.

Bone Broth

Bone broth, a powerhouse for your immune system, may help the body repair muscle tissue, cartilage, and ligaments, and assist with blood cell growth.[45] The collagen and other amino acids in bone broth will also make your hair and nails grow stronger, make your skin look better, help ease arthritis pain, and speed up the recovery of joint injuries.[46]

Bone broth is easy, although somewhat time-consuming, to make on your own. Simply place chicken or cow bones, preferably bones that have a lot of collagen and connective tissue, such as feet, wings, necks, and knuckles (in the case of cows) in a crockpot. Cover with water to the top, add ingredients such as carrots, celery, herbs, salt, pepper—whatever you like, for flavor. Then allow it to cook for at least 24 hours. The heat will break down the bones and all of the minerals and nutrients inside will go into the broth. A good quality bone broth will be very gelatinous. Gelatin is essentially cooked collagen, and collagen is particularly useful for healing skin and connective tissues. It's that sticky, gooey gelatin that you want to heal your gut walls.[47] I grew tired of making my own broth, and fortunately found a great product at Walmart, of all places. It is called Bonafide Provisions Bone Broth, and it is found in their organic freezer section. The cost is almost half the price of most other bone broths you may find at Whole Foods, and I find it is incredibly gelatinous.

Hydrolyzed Collagen

Yes, bone broth contains collagen. But, the collagen in bone broth is not as easily absorbed by the body as hydrolyzed collagen. Hydrolyzed collagen is partially broken down, so it's much easier for the body to metabolize and digest. Also, considering collagen is the second most plentiful substance in the human body, and that we produce less and less of it starting in our late 20's, it may make considerable sense to supplement with it.[48] There may also come a time when, like me, you simply tire of making bone broth or do not have access to it. Hydrolyzed collagen serves as your collagen insurance policy. I take it twice daily.

There are three sources of hydrolyzed collagen to consider: fish, beef, or chicken. Collagen is collagen, though, for the most part, so just ensure your hydrolyzed collagen powder is sourced from a healthy, humanely raised animal. Regardless of the animal source, collagen is essentially flavorless. Once you mix it with hot tea or coffee, you won't even know it's there.

I prefer a product called Great Lakes Gelatin Collagen Hydrolysate. It is excellent quality and mixes very well in hot beverages. Bulletproof Collagen is also a great choice. Be on the lookout, though, for products that add unnecessary junk like flavoring. Such ingredients are completely gratuitous and run counter to your reason for taking hydrolyzed collagen in the first place. *Always avoid added garbage*!

A Word About L-Glutamine in Supplement Form

While L-glutamine is good for you in a general sense, I firmly believe it should be taken in its natural form—from food, where it's in a suitable dose accompanied with other amino acids and nutrients your body needs.[49] Many well-intentioned functional medicine practitioners will recommend supplementing your diet with L-glutamine in pill or powder form. Some people do report good results with L-glutamine supplementation, but I personally would not take it in supplement form.

My experiences with L-glutamine supplementation demonstrated that it may cause potentially severe and unwanted side effects. I was encouraged to take L-glutamine to the tune of 10,000 mg daily divided into three doses. I was told it was completely safe, but if I was concerned, to start slowly and see how it affected me. I've always been quite sensitive to medicine and supplements, so I went slowly. After working up to just 2,000 mg once daily, I developed extreme neurological issues such that my eyes felt very heavy, and I found myself back in bed unable to function. It took several days for the effects to wear off.

Since this time, I've read that L-glutamine supplementation may be linked to cancer and may also contribute to the overgrowth of bad bugs in the gut.[50] I've also found scores of people on my Facebook Lyme disease forums who had neurological reactions similar to mine after taking this supplement. I suggest you proceed with caution if supplemental L-glutamine is recommended to you by any practitioner.

4. Fermented Foods

Fermentation has been used for hundreds of years as a natural way to preserve food. During the fermentation process, carbohydrates are converted to alcohol or organic acids using yeast or bacteria under anaerobic conditions.[51] The alcohol or acids in the fermentation process give the fermented food its characteristically zesty and tangy taste. Fermentation promotes the growth of beneficial bacteria, hence the many health benefits of fermented foods. Examples of fermented foods to enjoy are kefir, kombucha, sauerkraut, kimchi, beet kavas, and fermented pickles. I don't recommend store-bought yogurt, as it is a dairy product and typically loaded with sugar.

I recommend making your own fermented foods at home, particularly kefir. Kefir is a highly nutritious drink, loaded with beneficial bacteria, vitamins, minerals, amino acids, and compounds that can bolster your immune system.[52] Kefir is reported to contain up to 50 strains of probiotic bugs, making it the "mother" of all fermented foods. And, it's very easy and inexpensive to make. Simply purchase kefir grains on-line (I purchased mine from Amazon) and add a tablespoon to a half-gallon glass jar of goat milk or coconut milk. However, please note that coconut milk can be a bit temperamental to ferment, so I recommend finding a recipe especially for coconut milk kefir on-line. I avoid using cow milk entirely, as it causes me inflammation, likely due to its casein content. Goat milk does also contain casein, but it contains a type that is less apt to cause inflammation. Whether you choose goat or coconut milk, ensure the milk is full fat. There are recipes on-line for kefir, but the mechanics are the same. Cover the jar and allow it to sit on your counter for 24-48 hours, and voila! You've got kefir. I sometimes add probiotic capsules at the outset to ensure my kefir is absolutely loaded with beneficial bacteria. When it is done fermenting, I add cacao powder for taste. Check out this article for more recipes and information on the health benefits of kefir:

https://www.culturedfoodlife.com/7-reasons-i-have-kefir-every-day

You might be wondering why kefir, a dairy product (unless made with coconut milk), may be a healing food when dairy is generally prohibited in healing diets. One reason is that when milk is fermented, the bacteria turn the lactose in the milk into lactic acid. Enzymes in the kefir break the lactose down even further.[53] So, people who suffer from issues with dairy due to its lactose often have no problem whatsoever with kefir. The second reason is that goat milk kefir contains a type of casein that is less likely to cause inflammation than cow milk kefir. I always felt the healing properties of the beneficial bacteria in goat milk kefir outweighed my risks of inflammation. And, I never felt any negative reaction after drinking it. But again, everyone is different, so see how you feel after consuming kefir to know for sure.

Sauerkraut is also simple to make at home, and you can find endless recipes on-line. It's just as easy to make as kefir. Simply chop up cabbage, place in a large glass jar with water and salt, and let it sit and ferment for 5-7 days. I recommend finding a good recipe on-line, however, to ensure your end product is flavorful.

There really is no end to what you can ferment on your own, from pickles and beets to tea. If you can't ferment at home, most health-food stores now offer a wide variety of fermented foods such as kombucha, sauerkraut, fermented pickles, kimchi, and more. An excellent resource for fermenting food can be found at:

https://www.culturedfoodlife.com

There are certain situations, however, in which fermented foods may not be advisable, and I will discuss this in more depth later. If you know you suffer from histamine intolerance, small intestinal bacterial overgrowth (SIBO) or have an issue with candida, you may want to stay away from fermented foods until your problem is resolved. I tested positive for both candida and SIBO at the Cleveland Clinic. I also had issues with histamine. For a time, I was told by my practitioners to refrain from eating anything fermented. When I added fermented foods back into my diet, I went slowly and only ate them a few times per week. As you recover, you always want to monitor how you are reacting to anything you eat. If something seems to be giving you a problem, be flexible. Nothing is absolute when it comes to diet. There may be certain foods that your body simply cannot handle.

5. Healthy Fats

Finally, be sure to include healthy fats as a regular part of your diet. Fat is often demonized unnecessarily. Healthy fats, however, such as omega-3 and monounsaturated fats, are critical for energy production and cell growth and are an essential part of a healthy, balanced diet.[54] Sources of so-called healthy fats include fatty fish such as salmon (not farm-raised), walnuts, flaxseed, coconut oil, eggs (if you are not sensitive to them), nuts, and avocados.[55] When consuming nuts, it is advisable to soak them first in water overnight. Soaking breaks down phytic acid and enzyme inhibitors in the nuts, making them both easier to digest and more nutritious. Phytic acid can stop nutrients from being properly absorbed and diminish digestibility, while enzyme inhibitors can bind to nutrients, causing deficiencies and irritation in the digestive tract.[56]

Eating Healthy Made Easy—Smoothies!

I will share that the process of eating well became infinitely easier once I procured a Vitamix Blender. *The Wahls Protocol* calls for a fairly large amount of greens and colorful fruits and vegetables each day, and absent making a smoothie, I found it difficult to get everything into my meals. I also found that if I didn't have green drinks already made and readily available, I caved and ate whatever I could get my hands on. You certainly get hungrier when you are not eating an abundance of carbohydrates, so plan ahead. Having green drinks pre-made and ready to drink has been critical to my success.

About every other morning, I make a very large 64 ounce green smoothie using the Vitamix (and no, I am not paid to endorse this product!). I specifically use this blender because I've burned out the motors on almost every other brand of blender and learned the hard way that this one is worth its cost. The other benefit is taste. Take it from me, your green drinks will not be very palatable with any other blender. You will have chunks of pulp that will make you gag. My green drinks are absolutely packed with various greens, which I rotate each week. You want nice deep rich greens—not lettuce. I also add ginger root and various types of sulfur rich vegetables, such as broccoli or clover sprouts. To ensure I am getting my healthy fats, I add an entire avocado. You may want to add something like coconut milk—feel free to modify to suit your taste buds. Adding healthy fats to your smoothie is an easy way to work them into your diet. I then add approximately one cup of various frozen, low-sugar berries. Again, you want to continually rotate all of your fruits and vegetables to be sure you are getting a very nice variety of nutrients. The richer the color all the way through the fruit, the better. The equation is always essentially the same: heavy on the greens and lighter on the berries.

Once you've read *The Wahls Protocol*, you will have a solid grasp of how much of each ingredient to add to your smoothie. Your proportions will depend on how much you plan to drink in a day, as you want to ensure you get the daily requisite amount of greens, sulfur rich vegetables, and colorful vegetables and fruits. Once I've added all my vegetables and fruit, I fill it up with water, blend, and voila. I have four to five green drinks ready to go, which I then store in my refrigerator.

Please remember to use organic and properly cleaned fruits and vegetables. Water and vinegar with some baking soda work nicely to clean your fruits and vegetables.

Recommended Reading

The two books below are highly recommended as you get started honing your diet. The first book, *The Wahls Protocol*, is absolutely critical to your healing journey. The second book is optional, but is a fantastic resource for healing your gut, which as we've discussed, is fundamental to healing.

1. *The Wahls Protocol*, **by Dr. Terry Wahls**
2. *The Gut Health Protocol*, **by John G. Herron**

Remember, your body is unique to you, so your diet will need to be tweaked to meet your specific needs. These books will go into the detail necessary for you to finely tune your daily diet plan and regimen to fit your specific concerns. It is critical for you, as the "captain" of your recovery, to understand *why* what you eat matters. When you understand the "why" part, you will be much less likely to cheat and binge on a bag of potato chips. These books will help you better understand the science behind proper nutrition and supplementation, and the critical role food plays in cellular health.

Conclusion

Do you see a theme here? It should be clear by now that the crux to healing your gut and your body is to feed it only real, low-sugar, nutrient-dense food. If you can't grow it in your garden, kill it in the forest, or fish it out of the ocean, generally speaking, you shouldn't eat it. The body uses nutrients more readily when they are packaged and delivered in their natural state, so vitamin and mineral supplementation should not be the focus. Food is your medicine and primary source of vitamins and nutrients from this day forward. Don't question Mother Nature—she knows what she's doing.

Now, you may be asking, what is left to eat if bread, pasta, pizza, cereal, cheese, milk, and processed foods are forbidden? I will agree that it takes some adjusting to rid these things from your diet. But YOU are well worth the effort. If you don't clean up your diet, you may never get well. Once you dig in, you will find that there is an abundance of great tasting *real* food on this planet—the standard American diet is not all it's cracked up to be!

CHAPTER SEVEN

RECOVERY STEP #2—
Balance Your Hormones

*"Keep your face toward the sunshine and
shadows will fall behind you."*
Walt Whitman

Your hormones are often the first thing to fall out of whack when you're battling a chronic illness.[57] From energy levels to mood and sleep patterns, hormones play a critical role in our health or lack thereof.[58] Adrenal fatigue, thyroid disorders, anxiety, depression, histamine intolerance, and estrogen dominance or estrogen metabolism issues are all fairly common hormone-related problems seen in people with chronic illness, and their corresponding symptoms can be severely challenging.[59]

Estrogen's Link to Autoimmune Disease

Well worth noting is that 78% of those afflicted with autoimmune disease are women.[60] This strongly suggests a hormonal connection, namely estrogen, in the development of such illnesses.[61] It is believed that high estrogen may also reactivate viruses while reducing the immune system's ability to combat infection.[62] If you suffer from irregular menstrual cycles, thyroid disease, brain fog, endometriosis, insomnia, or fatigue, you may have estrogen dominance, or an inability to properly metabolize estrogen.[63] Addressing hormonal imbalances, particularly estrogen, may be a critical step in your recovery. An experienced functional medicine practitioner can help you sort these problems out.

When I look back on my life, I realize I have been symptomatic of estrogen imbalance since my early teens. As a teenager, I had fairly severe and recurrent bouts of anxiety and depression. Then, in my twenties, I developed endometriosis. Add to this, I was raised on the standard American diet with the belief that a bowl of processed, sugar-coated cereal and a Flintstone's Vitamin represented a healthy start to the day. It certainly is not difficult to see where the cracks in my foundation originated.

If you suspect you have problems with estrogen but are not able to see a functional medicine practitioner, there are estrogen saliva tests you can take at home. Although remember, these tests only provide a snapshot of one moment in time, and therefore, are only so reliable. For approximately $85, I tested my estrogen levels using the ZRT Laboratory Estrogen Dominance Saliva Home Test. It was very simple to administer and confirmed what I'd already suspected.

Adrenal Fatigue

Anyone suffering from a chronic illness may also suffer from adrenal fatigue. The adrenal glands are small triangular shaped glands located on top of both kidneys that produce various hormones to help regulate metabolism, the immune system, blood pressure, and the body's stress response.[64] If you feel tired and run down, your adrenal glands may be overworked and not functioning properly.[65]

Dr. James L. Wilson, the authority on adrenal fatigue, defines the condition as:

> [A] deficiency in the functioning of the adrenal glands. Normally functioning adrenal glands secrete minute, yet precise and balanced amounts of steroid hormones. But because they are designed to be so very responsive to changes in your inner physical, emotional and psychological environment, any number of factors can interfere with this finely tuned balance. This means that too much physical, emotional, environmental, and/or psychological stress can deplete your adrenals, causing a decrease in the output of adrenal hormones, particularly cortisol. This lowered adrenal activity (hypoadrenia), resulting from adrenal fatiue, can range in severity all the way from almost zero to almost normal.[66]

Symptoms of Adrenal Fatigue May Include:[67]

1. Fatigue upon waking that is not relieved by more sleep
2. Craving for salty foods
3. Lethargy
4. Increased effort to complete everyday tasks
5. Decreased productivity
6. Decreased ability to handle stress
7. Increased time to recover from illness, injury, or trauma
8. Light-headedness upon standing
9. Mild depression
10. Less enjoyment or happiness with life
11. Increased PMS
12. Increased symptoms with skipped or inadequate meals
13. Brain fog
14. Memory problems
15. Afternoon energy low between 3:00 and 4:00 PM

16. Improved symptoms after evening meal

So, how do you heal burned out adrenal glands? It is not a simple answer. It's been my experience that as my overall health improved, my adrenal health also improved. And quite tellingly, according to most experts in this area, healing the adrenal glands requires a proper diet, as outlined herein, getting plenty of sleep each night (sleeping in until at least 8:30 AM if possible as those last few hours in the morning are when Dr. Wilson states the adrenal glands heal the most), reducing your stress load, practicing mindfulness and meditation, and using some targeted supplementation. The adaptogenic herbs recommended for adrenal health have broad ranging effects that will not only help your adrenal glands but will fight infection and reduce systemic inflammation.

For an in-depth discussion on adrenal fatigue, I recommend reading Dr. Wilson's book, *Adrenal Fatigue The 21st Century Stress Syndrome*. Dr. Wilson provides a wealth of information and recommendations on how to overcome adrenal fatigue if this is a stubborn problem for you. Dr. Wilson also developed a line of supplements for adrenal health and these can be purchased on-line.

My Favorite Supplements for Adrenal Health Include:

1. **Ashwagandha**
   Ashwagandha is an adaptogenic herb, meaning it may help the body balance hormones that are either too high or too low. It's an ancient medicinal herb that has been used for over 3,000 years to relieve stress, and increase energy and concentration.[68] Among its many reported benefits, ashwagandha may help lower cortisol levels, exhibit anti-cancer properties, reduce blood sugar levels, and reduce inflammation.[69] Its impact on cortisol is what makes it particularly useful in adrenal fatigue, as taxed adrenal glands get stuck in a chronic state of excess cortisol production.

If you can't sleep at night, cortisol could be the problem and ashwagandha may help.

2. **Holy Basil**
Holy basil has been referred to as both the "Queen of Herbs" and the "elixir of life."[70] It is definitely one of my favorite adaptogenic herbs, and it has a broad range of benefits. Holy basil may be very helpful in relieving stress and anxiety, in restoring sleep, improving memory and cognition, improving digestion, and alleviating inflammation while also being antimicrobial, anti-viral, and anti-fungal.[71] It is said to help stabilize blood sugar, which is critical for balancing hormones, while also helping the liver to detox excess hormones to prevent estrogen dominance.[72]

3. **HPA Adapt by Integrative Therapeutics**
This product combines several adaptogenic herbs to assist the body with a proper stress response. The herbs in this product include rhodiola, ashwagandha, eleuthero, holy basil, and maca. This particular supplement contains arguably the best adaptogenic herbs that exist in nature. It may help not only with adrenal fatigue, but also with menopause and PMS.

A word of caution, however. Maca, rhodiola, and eleuthero may negatively impact estrogen levels. People who are estrogen dominant, or slow to metabolize estrogen, could have a poor response to these herbs.[73] It truly is a trial and error process, so always go slowly. There is a lot of literature on the positive impacts of maca, for instance, on balancing hormones, and many sources claim it balances estrogen. My practitioner, however, told me that in his practice patients sometimes have negative reactions to maca, and he suspects it may slow the metabolization of estrogen in some women. Yet another reason why it's always optimal to work with a qualified practitioner when dealing in herbs.

If you have endometriosis and known estrogen issues, you may simply want to take adaptogenic herbs individually so you know how you react. Ashwagandha and holy basil are two great places in my opinion to start. I have taken these two herbs for long periods of time to balance my hormones with great results.

4. **Vital Plan Adaptogen Recovery**

   Vital Plan makes an excellent product called Adaptogen Recovery, which combines several adaptogenic herbs into one product. It contains Chinese skullcap, cordyceps, reishi mushroom, and rehmannia. Each of these ingredients may be beneficial to adrenal health and may support a proper stress response in the body.[74]

5. **Vitamin C**

   Vitamin C is found in high concentrations in the adrenal glands and can become depleted when we are stressed.[75] Vitamin C is not only critical for the proper functioning of our adrenal glands, but it also helps manage cortisol levels. Food sources of vitamin C include fruits and vegetables that are bright in color such as citrus fruits, peppers, cauliflower and broccoli. But when you suffer adrenal fatigue or immune challenges, these sources of vitamin C may not be enough. I have supplemented with two types of vitamin C with great success. One is called Lypo-Spheric Vitamin C by LivOn Laboratories. It is a lyposomal vitamin C, and is purported to be very highly absorbable. The other product I use is called Effer-C by Douglas Laboratories.

6. **Stress B-Complex by Thorne**

   B vitamins are also critical for the repair and proper functioning of our adrenal glands.[76] When choosing a vitamin B supplement, it's important to ensure it is a methylated complex. It is estimated that approximately 30% of the population may be unable to properly metabolize certain B vitamins, specifically folate and Vitamin B12.[77] The methylated form ensures your body will metabolize the vitamins, so you will not be wasting your money or contributing to a problem. If you are unable to metabolize folate, for instance (a condition known as MTHFR gene mutation), it can build up in your system and create negative side effects. Thorne Stress B-Complex is formulated for proper absorption and has the proper ratio of the B vitamins taxed adrenal glands may need. Pure Encapsulations is another company that makes a high quality vitamin B supplement.

Thyroid Disease

Thyroid problems are quite common in women, particularly those with chronic illness. They can be very tricky to resolve, and you should work with a practitioner if you suffer any sort of thyroid condition. That said, there is a lot you can do on your own to improve your thyroid health. And I know this, because I did it.

At the height of my illness, I was diagnosed as having an autoimmune thyroid. My thyroid blood scores showed I had elevated antibodies, but my thyroid hormones were still in the normal range. I also had a small goiter and several nodules on my thyroid gland. Technically, my doctor said I had Hashimoto's disease, but my thyroid was apparently still pumping out the right amount of hormones. He said eventually, though, my thyroid gland would stop doing this because of the autoimmune attack. His solution was to put me on Synthroid, which he said I would be on for life. According to my doctor at the time, no one knew why Hashimoto's disease occurred, but once it did, it was a lifelong condition and Synthroid was the answer. Not knowing any better or having any understanding of the impact a proper nutrient-dense diet could have on my health, I believed him and took Synthroid.

Synthroid made me feel absolutely horrible. I was already very sick from everything else going wrong in my body, but this took it to a new level.

I threw the Synthroid in the garbage and immediately dove headfirst into researching thyroid disease. The first thing I learned was that diet is critical, as is the case with any autoimmune problem. The second thing I learned was that there are supplements that can potentially stop the autoimmune attack on my thyroid gland.

I'm not going to dive too far into a discussion on thyroid disease, because it is a very complicated topic. But I will give you the nuts and bolts of what helped me, so that you can get on the correct path.

First and foremost, if you are suffering from a thyroid condition, I highly recommend the following two books to help you with your treatment plan.

1. *Stop the Thyroid Madness*, **by Janie A. Bowethorpe, M.Ed.**
2. *Why Do I Still Have Thyroid Symptoms*, **by Dr. Datis Kharrazian.**

These two books will answer all of your questions, and then some, on thyroid health and how to restore it.

One supplement in particular that helped me was Thytrophin PMG by Standard Process. According to my functional medicine practitioner, this supplement acts as a shield around the thyroid gland, protecting it from autoimmune attacks. It contains bovine thyroid PMG extract processed to remove thyroxine thyroid hormone.[78] It may be able to impact your thyroid hormone levels, so as always, work with a practitioner if possible. For me, my thyroid scores were not impacted, but my antibody levels went back to normal. There are other herbal supplements you can work into your regimen to support thyroid health, and these are discussed thoroughly in the two aforementioned books.

Diet was the other missing link for me. Once I removed gluten, grains, and processed sugar and identified the foods that caused my body inflammation, my thyroid problems slowly improved. As Dr. Wahls explains so well in her book, *The Wahls Protocol*, autoimmune disease is simply your immune system run amok. You need to throw water on the fire and calm the body down. That will mean determining which foods are causing you inflammation and making your immune system go into overdrive. You can do this by implementing an elimination diet and/or by having a blood test done to determine which foods are giving you an immune response.

How do you know if you have a thyroid condition? If you have one or more symptoms from the list below, it is quite possible.[79] See your doctor for testing and be sure he or she is not just measuring your TSH levels. To truly know the health of your thyroid gland, you will ideally have a full blood panel run, which includes TbAb and Anti-Tpo (antibodies), TSH, T3, free T3, T4, free T4 and reverse T3. You may also need an ultrasound image to detect nodules or a goiter.

Common Symptoms of Thyroid Disease Include:[80]

1. Fatigue
2. Cold sensitivity / cold hands or feet
3. Feeling too hot
4. Constipation
5. Dry skin
6. Weight gain
7. Puffy face
8. Hoarseness
9. Muscle weakness
10. Dry or brittle hair or hair loss
11. Memory problems
12. Irritability or depression
13. High cholesterol
14. Slower heart rate

Anxiety & Depression

Battling a chronic and debilitating illness is reason enough to suffer anxiety and depression. I was often asked by my practitioners if I was depressed or anxious, and I'd look at them like, *what do you think?* Of course I was! Anyone would be under the same circumstances. I knew, however, if my circumstances changed overnight, and I found myself with completely restored health, that my anxiety and depression would be a thing of the past. In other words, it was almost entirely situational.

You may find, though, that your mood starts to become something less about your situation and more about a chemical imbalance. When you're sick for an extended period of time, unable to exercise or socialize as you once did, it's quite understandable that the brain could fall off balance. True depression is something much different than simply being upset about your current state of affairs. If you suffer true clinical depression, please see a doctor to determine the proper course of action.

As I noted earlier in this book, scientists have discovered that almost 90% of the brain's serotonin is produced in the gut.[81] Serotonin is the key hormone usually deficient in people with anxiety and depression. If you are chronically ill, your gut is likely in rough shape. Your depression and anxiety may resolve, or at least improve, once you improve your gut health. This requires that you overhaul your diet, implement a proper herbal protocol, improve your sleep, and begin to exercise again. Exercise, which I discuss in more depth in Chapter 11, will also boost "feel good" hormones, such as dopamine and serotonin. In particular, many of the herbs I discussed for adrenal fatigue can be very beneficial for alleviating anxiety and depression.

My Favorite Supplements for Anxiety and Depression Include:

1. **Ashwaghanda**
   As previously discussed, this adaptogenic herb has worked wonderfully for me in curbing anxiety and improving my sleep patterns by keeping my cortisol levels in proper range. Because this herb helps to normalize stress hormones, such as adrenaline and cortisol, it may help improve your mood and ability to handle stress.[82]

2. **Holy Basil**
   Similar to ashwaghanda, this adaptogenic herb has also been very helpful in bringing my hormones into balance and restoring my sleep. This powerful herb is said to have antidepressant and anti-anxiety properties similar to those found with antidepressant drugs.[83]

3. **B-Complex Plus by Pure Encapsulations**
   B vitamins may be very helpful in curbing anxiety and depression, as they help the nervous system to operate smoothly.[84] As stated earlier, it is important to select a methylated B vitamin complex to ensure proper absorption. Pure Encapsulations B-Complex Plus is well regarded by practitioners and provides B vitamins in their proper methylated form.

4. **Natural Calm Plus Calcium by Natural Vitality**
   This product is a blend of magnesium citrate, vitamins C & D, calcium, potassium, and boron. I found it particularly helpful in settling down heart palpitations and helping me relax for sleep. Getting restorative and regular sleep is critical to balancing hormones, and, therefore, in curbing anxiety and depression.

As always, work with a medical doctor and functional medicine practitioner, if possible, on these issues. But rest assured, your depression and anxiety will likely improve or resolve once you strictly implement a gut healing diet, proper exercise regimen, and follow the principles outlined in this book.

Histamine Intolerance & Estrogen Metabolism

Histamine is a neurotransmitter that aids the body with many functions, namely in helping to identify toxins or foreign invaders. When the body creates histamine, the result is inflammation.[85] If you have seasonal allergies, you will quickly identify with the runny nose and red itchy eyes that histamines create. This immune response helps your white blood cells find the issue inside the body and resolve it. Enzymes will then break down the histamine.[86] But what happens if your body cannot properly break down histamine? In some people, histamine may build up in the body and create a host of symptoms from fatigue and skin rashes to dizziness and migraines.[87]

I found out I had a problem with histamine the hard way. I broke out in a very painful, head-to-toe rash after a meal. A few days later, when it hadn't resolved and my body was blowing up like a balloon in all directions, I ended up in the emergency room. My reaction persisted for almost four months.

At my initial exam, the allergy doctor asked if I'd had any unusual hot flashes lately. I wasn't sure where she was going with the question or what a hot flash might have to do with my problem. I simply told her I was not experiencing hot flashes. On my drive home, reflecting upon her question, it dawned on me that I'd been having an endometriosis flair leading up to this allergic reaction. I'd been diagnosed with endometriosis many years earlier, in 2002, and I've dealt with cysts for many years. Estrogen fluctuations may drive the formation of cysts and endometriosis. Estrogen fluctuations may also drive hot flashes.

Turns out, estrogen may also increase histamine. Histamine then stimulates the production of more estrogen.[88] Estrogen also down-regulates diamine oxidase (DAO), which the body uses to break down histamines.[89] Put these puzzle pieces together, and you have a wicked cycle of too much histamine floating around with no means of escape. I suspect in my situation, my heightened endometriosis symptoms meant my estrogen levels were off, which negatively impacted my ability to break down histamine.

So, what do you do in this situation? First, you want to address any issues with estrogen dominance or metabolism. I did this by adding DIM, a supplement that assists with proper estrogen metabolism, to my rotation as well as ensuring strict adherence to *The Wahls Protocol* diet. Second, you can use targeted supplementation to assist the body in properly breaking down histamine. Below, I have listed the supplements I found most helpful. Third, you can avoid histamine rich foods, but this will put you on an extremely restrictive diet.[90] A quick Google search will show you the nearly never-ending list of histamine rich foods, including fermented food, avocados, cheese, bananas, nuts, lemons, vinegar, bone broth, and chocolate. I cut back on foods I knew were *very* high in histamines, such as nuts, anything fermented, and dark chocolate. But aside from that, I let it go. I wanted to stick with my healthy, nutrient-dense diet that would heal my gut—the ultimate histamine intolerance solution—and I wasn't going to tax myself stressing over whether each food I ate contained high amounts of histamine.

Supplements That May Relieve Histamine Intolerance & Improve Estrogen Metabolism:[91]

1. **DAO**

    Diamine oxidase, discussed above, which breaks down histamines in the body.

2. **Quercetin**

   A plant pigment found in vegetables such as onions, it may help the body break down histamines.

3. **DIM**

   Naturally found in broccoli and cabbage, it may help the body properly regulate estrogen levels. This in turn may help to keep histamine at a proper level.[92]

4. **Ancestral Supplements Kidney**

   Essentially ground up kidney, an organ meat, a natural source of DAO.

Supplementation requires trial and error, as there are many decent products out there to help with breaking down histamine and excess estrogen. It all depends on which ones work for you. Over time and with much patience, I saw my histamine issues settle down.

Much has been written on histamine intolerance, and *The Gut Health Protocol*, by John Herron, delves more deeply into this topic. The internet is also an excellent resource if you are experiencing histamine issues or suspect you are experiencing them. As with anything, there is no magic-bullet solution, and the best place to start is with your diet. Determining which foods give you a reaction is critical.

This also serves as an excellent reminder that just because a food is technically "healthy," does not mean it is healthy *for you*! The weird symptoms you've been experiencing for years might be due to a histamine problem.

A Quick Word On Endometriosis

For female readers who also struggle with endometriosis and do not want to treat it with prescription drugs, I use two different over-the-counter products called SerraRx by Biomedic Labs and Serracor-NK by AST

Enzymes. When taken together three times a day on an empty stomach, these supplements have been incredibly effective for me in resolving endometriosis pain and dissolving cysts. I also take DIM, which is naturally found in broccoli and cabbage, and may help regulate estrogen levels.[93] Ashwagandha and holy basil, two of my favorite adaptogenic herbs for balancing hormones, may also be very helpful in curbing endometriosis symptoms.

Conclusion

Correcting a hormonal imbalance takes time and patience. Unfortunately, it requires a lot of trial and error, as some modalities work for some but not others. Results will not likely come overnight, but will instead unfold slowly over time as you commit to your diet plan and protocol. If your hormonal imbalances are particularly stubborn or involve your thyroid, it is advisable to work with a practitioner who can administer blood tests and give you targeted advice.

CHAPTER EIGHT

RECOVERY STEP #3— Combat Infection with Targeted Herbal Protocols

"Let your faith be bigger than your fear."
Hebrews 13:6

The next critical step in repairing your gut and improving your health is to knock out any overgrowth of bad bugs and/or parasites. I accomplished this with a low-sugar diet and herbal antimicrobials. There are endless herbal protocols to choose from. The great thing about herbs is that they will not destroy your beneficial bacteria, but rather will work slowly and stealth-like to eradicate the bad guys. And, very importantly, you can take most herbs for prolonged periods. So, you can use them as an insurance policy to maintain your health long after you've recovered. That's an enormous benefit that does not come with antibiotics. Not to mention that certain herbs have a tremendously synergistic effect when taken together and can help improve all areas of your health.

Many herbal protocols market themselves specifically to Lyme disease sufferers. But, if Lyme is not your specific problem, I don't feel that should stop you from taking them. If you suffer from any chronic condition, you almost certainly have an overgrowth of bad bugs in your gut. And even if you don't, herbs tend to be broad ranging in their impact. They not only make your body inhospitable to all sorts of infection (not just Lyme), but they can boost your immune system in significant ways and help your body to get well and stay well.

In other words, you are quite unlikely to hurt yourself taking an herbal protocol (provided you follow the dosing instructions properly), and the benefits can be substantial. In fact, one of the doctors I consulted with who recovered from his own chronic health problems using herbs, told me he continues to follow his herbal protocols now that he's well. And incredibly, as he sticks to his herbal remedies, his health continually gets better and better each year. He reported feeling better in his 50s than he did in his 30s when he was allegedly healthy!

My Favorite Herbal Protocols

1. Cowden
2. Zhang
3. Stephen Buhner
4. Vital Plan Restore Kit

1. Cowden Protocol

The Cowden Protocol was developed by Dr. Lee Cowden, a retired cardiologist in Dallas, Texas. Dr. Cowden successfully treated a patient suffering from chronic Lyme disease with herbs after he failed to respond to antibiotic therapies. The patient recovered, and the Cowden Protocol was born. The Cowden Protocol incorporates a large number of herbs over a long period of time. There is also a modified Cowden Protocol that uses only a handful of herbs at a fraction of the price. But, obviously, such an abbreviated protocol will not be nearly as effective on stubborn or acute infection.

Cowden Protocol Herbs Include:

1. Banderol
2. Samento
3. Burbur
4. Cumanda
5. Amantilla
6. Enula
7. Houttuynia
8. Mora
9. Magnesium Malate
10. Parsley
11. Pinella
12. Sealantro
13. Stevia
14. Takuna
15. Serrapeptase

Modified Cowden Protocol Herbs Include:

1. Samento
2. Banderol
3. Cumanda
4. Burbur

The full Cowden Protocol takes anywhere from five to nine months to complete at a cost of approximately $350 per month. A calendar spreadsheet comes with the program that maps out precisely when and how to take each herbal tincture. The modified program is obviously much less expensive, as it requires only a select core group of herbs. Generally speaking, these herbs are taken three times per day in one ounce of water, working up to thirty drops of each delineated herb per day. If money is an issue, the modified protocol is a good place to start. The Cowden Protocol can be purchased at: www.nutramedix.com.

2. The Zhang Protocol

Dr. Qingcai Zhang is a doctor from New York City who has successfully treated chronic infections for the past fifty years. Dr. Zhang is particularly adept with treating Lyme disease using Chinese medicine. Dr. Zhang's protocol combines specific herbs for a broad approach to tackling infection.[94] The herbs used in Dr. Zhang's Protocol support the body's immune system and natural detoxification processes while making it difficult for an infection to survive.

Many people report having success with the Zhang Protocol when antibiotics and traditional therapies have failed. Dr. Zhang's herbs are, however, quite expensive. Dr. Darin Ingel provides an excellent spreadsheet on-line outlining how to effectively administer Dr. Zhang's herbs. His pdf presentation entitled, "Identifying and Resolving The Lyme Paradox," can be found at:

https://restorativemedicine.org/wpcontent/uploads/2017/01/11Ingels_Lyme-Paradox.pdf

I highly recommend the Zhang Protocol if it is within your financial means. If not, do not fret. There are many ways to skin a cat.

Herbs in the Zhang Protocol Include:

1. Artemisiae (contains wormwood, astragalus, and codonopsis)
2. Houttuynia
3. Circulation P (two formulas with combination of ten Chinese herbs)
4. Coptis

5. Cordyceps
6. Puerania
7. R-5081 (smilax glabra root, Baikai skullcap root, Chinese goldthread rhizome, dandelion, Japanese honeysuckle flower, Polygoni cuspidate rhizome, and Chinese licorice root)
8. AI#3 (Macunae caulis, Sargentodoxae caulis, Paederiae caulis)
9. Allicin

3. Stephen Buhner Protocol

Herbalist Stephen Buhner is considered an authority on Lyme disease, as his herbal recommendations have been very effective in combatting chronic infection. Buhner has authored more than twenty books on the healing properties of herbs. In particular, I recommend, *"Healing Lyme,"* and *"Healing Lyme Disease Co-infections,"* both available for purchase on-line.

Buhner Protocol Herbs Include:

1. Japanese knotwood
2. Cat's claw
3. Andrographis

There are numerous other herbs included in Buhner's protocols and these are outlined in depth in his books.

4. Vital Plan Restore Kit

Dr. William Rahls was an obstetrician practicing in North Carolina when he fell sick with Lyme disease in 2003. He struggled for years with mysterious symptoms, going from doctor to doctor as most of us do, to find a diagnosis. After conventional medicine failed him, Dr. Rahls turned to herbal remedies to heal his chronic illness. He went on to develop his own herbal protocol inspired in part by herbalist Stephen

Buhner. Ultimately, Dr. Rahls took all that he learned from his years practicing medicine and recovering from illness to develop the Vital Plan Restore Kit.

The Vital Plan Restore Kit can be purchased on-line at: www.vitalplan.com. Along with the Restore Kit, Dr. Rahls has developed an extensive line of individual herbal supplements to help the body recover from chronic disease and maintain wellness once health has been restored.

Dr. Rahls has assembled some of the best synergistic herbs into his products. My only critique of his product line is that some of the dosages seem conservatively low, in my opinion. Overall though, I've found his products to be helpful, and his staff is quite responsive to questions by both phone and email. Dr. Rahls also offers excellent webinars on a regular basis where you can ask questions about your specific health challenges and get more detailed information as to how to use his products.

Very Honorable Mention Herbal Protocols

Of course, the four herbal protocols listed above are not the only protocols to choose from. Below, I list other top herbal protocols that you may want to look into. I did not use these protocols very extensively, but they come highly recommended by practitioners. I've also read very positive user reviews from other Lyme disease sufferers as to their effectiveness.

1. **Dr. David Jernigan, DC** – Dr. Jernigan carries a line of herbal products designed to combat Lyme disease and chronic illness. His products can be purchased on-line. For more information, visit Dr. Jernigan's web site at www.biologixcenter.com.

2. **Beyond Balance** – Susan McCamish developed a line of herbal tinctures for chronic Lyme disease and chronic illness. Her products

are very well regarded and widely used. For more information, visit www.beyondbalance.com.

3. **Byron White Formulas** – these herbal tinctures are also used for chronic Lyme disease and other chronic illnesses. They are available through licensed practitioners. For more information, visit www.byronwhiteformulas.com.

Individual Antimicrobial Foods & Supplements

If for some reason you do not wish to tackle an extensive herbal protocol that involves multiple products at once, you should, at a minimum, incorporate specific antimicrobial foods and/or one or two (or three) antimicrobial supplements into your rotation.

The antimicrobial foods and supplements discussed below are fairly regular staples in my routine. With the exception of apple cider vinegar and baking soda, I do not take them every day, but I have them readily available. Some supplements, such as CandiBactin-AR and CandiBactin-BR, I've taken for extended periods if symptoms warranted, per my practitioner.

My Favorite "Stand-Alone" Antimicrobial Foods & Supplements:

1. Apple Cider Vinegar with Baking Soda
2. Sovereign Silver
3. CandiBactin-AR & CandiBactin-BR
4. Advanced Biotic by Vital Plan
5. Monolaurin
6. Effer C by Douglas Laboratories
7. Cayennade Kombucha by GT's
8. Pumpkin Seeds
9. Diatomaceous Earth ("DE")
10. Microbe Formulas Full Moon Kit

1. Apple Cider Vinegar with Baking Soda

Both apple cider vinegar and baking soda are believed to have many health benefits. Apple cider vinegar is purported to lower blood sugar and cholesterol, while also being antibacterial and possibly even having anti-cancer effects.[95] Baking soda on the other hand, is a purported remedy for intestinal parasites, gout (by preventing the formation of uric acid crystals), and may also be antiviral, antifungal, and antibacterial.[96] Quite interestingly, it was recently reported that baking soda can also help calm the inflammatory response in autoimmune disease. As reported in Science Daily:

> *"Drinking baking soda ... tells the spleen...to go easy on the immune response. Certainly drinking bicarbonate affects the spleen and we think it's through the mesothelial cells," O'Connor says. The conversation, which occurs with the help of the chemical messenger acetylcholine, appears to promote a landscape that shifts against inflammation, they report.*[97]

> *In the spleen, as well as the blood and kidneys, they found after drinking water with baking soda for two weeks, the population of immune cells called macrophages, shifted from primarily those that promote inflammation, called M1, to those that reduce it, called M2. Macrophages, perhaps best known for their ability to consume garbage in the body like debris from injured or dead cells, are early arrivers to a call for an immune response.*[98]

If I feel a cold or virus coming on, I will take a tablespoon or so of apple cider vinegar with ¼ teaspoon of baking soda and some water on an empty stomach three times per day. As a maintenance dose, I take this once daily. The combination of these two ingredients is believed to create an alkaline environment in the body, making it less hospitable to infection and disease.[99] I find that the combination of apple cider vinegar and baking soda helps me fend off colds and viruses like nothing else. Have some food handy after the apple cider vinegar and baking soda mixture goes down, as it can upset your stomach.

Please be somewhat cautious with baking soda. Because it is salt, it has the potential to impact your blood pressure. If you have high blood pressure, you will want to consult your doctor before adding it to your regimen.

2. Sovereign Silver

Sovereign Silver is purported to act like a natural antibiotic, and is therefore recommended by functional medicine practitioners for bacterial infections. Many practitioners use Sovereign Silver for Lyme disease, either alone or in conjunction with antibiotics. It can be purchased online at retailers such as Amazon or at local health food stores. A little goes a long way with this product, so always follow the dosage guidelines per the bottle. I have used Sovereign Silver successfully for strep throat, and I also take it any time I feel a symptom brewing. You can take this product in conjunction with apple cider vinegar and baking soda for a one-two punch.

3. CandiBactin-AR and CandiBactin-BR by Metagenics

My Cleveland Clinic practitioner claimed her patients achieved excellent results with these two products taken together, and I was no exception. I found both supplements to be excellent for combatting candida overgrowth and small intestinal bacterial overgrowth (SIBO). They are expensive, but they worked for me. CandiBactin-AR is a concentrated blend of essential oils including thyme, oregano, sage, and lemon balm.[100] CandiBactin-BR contains coptis, oregon grape, berberine HCL, Chinese skullcap, phellodendron bark, ginger rhizome, Chinese licorice root, and Chinese rhubarb root and rhizome.[101]

4. Advanced Biotic by Vital Plan

This product is affordable and contains a nice assortment of antimicrobial herbs. It's a broad range herbal product that includes Japanese knotweed, cat's claw, andrographis, garlic, sarsaparilla, and berberine. From my understanding on herbal remedies, however, the dosages may be conservative for combatting a Lyme infection or anything acute. You can contact Vital Plan to discuss altering the recommended dosage based on your health concerns, or of course, discuss directly with your healthcare provider.

5. Monolaurin

Monolaurin is an excellent anti-viral supplement. I personally prefer Ecological Formulas brand, but many practitioners recommend Lauricidin brand. My functional medicine practitioner noted that monolaurin may be particularly effective at combatting Epstein Barre Syndrome when taken at higher dosages of about 3-5000mg per day in divided doses. For a maintenance dose (per my practitioner), about 1800mg is sufficient to combat the common cold or other viruses floating around during cold and flu season.

6. Effer C by Douglas Laboratories

This is a powerful buffered vitamin C supplement that was recommended to me by my naturopath to use during cold and flu season, although I use it year-round. It contains 1,175mg of vitamin C, 225mg calcium, 125mg magnesium ascorbate/oxide, and 49.5mg of potassium. I find that this vitamin C is highly effective at helping me get over a cold quickly or conversely at preventing me from getting sick. Vitamin C is noted to have powerful antibacterial and antiviral effects, so it is extremely helpful for anyone with a compromised immune system and chronic illness.

7. Cayennade Kombucha by GT's

This fermented beverage has been incredibly effective for me in fighting viruses. This kombucha contains cayenne pepper, ginger, and lemon. It's very hot, but that's likely why it works! When I feel a sore throat or a cold coming on, I drink this throughout the day. I've staved off a number of colds using this beverage, and probably the flu. Being a mom, when my kids come down with a stomach bug, I end up in the trenches with them. This past year, I drank this kombucha specifically twice daily when my daughter was home with stomach flu and managed to avoid getting sick. This beverage is a bit high in sugar, however, so don't over-do it. I generally would not consume more than one 16oz bottle in divided doses per day.

8. Pumpkin Seeds

Pumpkin seeds pack a big punch in a small body. They are a great source of antioxidants, magnesium, iron, and zinc.[102] They also contain high levels of cucurbitins, a substance that can paralyze intestinal parasites and worms so your body can properly expel them.[103] People with chronic health problems are often unwitting hosts to parasites that are difficult to diagnose. Pumpkin seeds can help ensure you are not one of those hosts! Simply take ½ cup of pumpkin seeds, blend them well (use your Vitamix if you have one) with ½ cup coconut or almond milk and ½ cup water.[104] The end result should be a bit pasty, and you eat it like you would oatmeal or porridge.[105]

9. Diatomaceous Earth ("DE")

Diatomaceous earth, or DE, is made up of the fossilized remains of diatoms, which are a type of algae found in river and lake beds.[106] The cell walls of these diatoms are made of silica and they easily break down into a fine powder. DE is said to kill parasites and viruses while cleaning the digestive tract, improving liver function, and absorbing harmful chemicals in the blood.[107] You must be sure that your DE is food grade, however, before ingesting. It is easy to take, simply add a teaspoon to a tablespoon in water and drink once daily. If using the pumpkin seed paste recipe presented above for parasites, it is recommended to follow it up with DE and plenty of water.[108]

10. Microbe Formulas Full Moon Kit

Microbe Formulas offer three herbal products meant to be taken together for a 3, 5, or 7 day parasite and pathogen cleanse. Many people report incredible results with this cleanse, and it is easy and affordable to complete. For more information on how this cleanse works, or to purchase the cleanse, visit: www.microbeformulas.com.

Antimicrobials for Treating SIBO & SIFO

Small intestinal bacterial overgrowth (SIBO) and small intestinal fungal overgrowth (SIFO) are two fairly common gastrointestinal problems found in people suffering from chronic illness. These conditions occur when an excess amount of either bacteria or fungus (typically candida or yeast) grow in the small intestine, creating moderate to sometimes very severe gastrointestinal issues and other symptoms.[109] The main cause of SIBO is typically anything that causes blockages or a slowdown in gut flow. The small intestine is supposed to be relatively devoid of bacteria, as its main job is to break food down and absorb nutrients.[110] When the food you ate sits in the small intestines partially broken down, it feeds bacteria. Before long, you will have dysbiosis in your small intestine and symptoms such as bloating and gas.

How do you know if you have SIBO or SIFO? Your practitioner can perform a breath test for SIBO. Life Extension also sells a SIBO Home Breath Kit that you can purchase on-line and take in the comfort of your own home. Currently, there are no simple breath tests available for SIFO. You can, however, determine the likelihood of having either SIBO or SIFO by taking a survey of symptoms.

Common SIBO & SIFO Symptoms:[111]

1. Gas, bloating, diarrhea, constipation, or cramping
2. Unexplained weight loss or weight gain
3. Fatigue
4. Currently suffer an autoimmune illness such as Hashimoto's, lupus, fibromyalgia, or CFS
5. Brain fog
6. Acne, psoriasis, eczema, or hives
7. Mood swings, anxiety, depression, or panic disorder
8. Frequent infections, especially UTIs, vaginal infections, or ear infections
9. Sugar and carb cravings
10. Seasonal allergies
11. Food intolerances
12. Vitamin B12 deficiency

What else should you do if you suspect SIBO or SIFO? First, you need to modify your diet to ensure you are eliminating excess sugars and starchy carbohydrates. Practitioners typically recommend a low FODMAP diet as your first course of action.[112] FODMAP is an acronym for Fermentable Oligosaccharides, Disaccharides, Monosaccharides, and Polyols. These are specific carbohydrates that may not be easily broken down, and therefore they will sit and enable bacteria to grow.[113] The low FODMAP diet is very restrictive and should only be followed for a short period of time.

A quick Google search will give you access to charts outlining precisely what foods are permissible on a low FODMAP diet. There are simply too many foods to list here, and frankly, the charts available on-line are excellent. One such web-site that offers pdf charts outlining the details of the FODMAP diet can be found at: https://www.dietvsdisease.org/diy-low-fodmap-diet.

Examples of High FODMAP Foods to Avoid:[114]

1. Onions
2. Brocolli
3. Cabbage
4. Cauliflower
5. Snow peas
6. Asparagus
7. Artichokes
8. Brussel sprouts
9. Mushrooms
10. Celery
11. Sweet Corn
12. Peaches
13. Apricots
14. Nectarines
15. Apples
16. Blackberries
17. Dairy products containing lactose
18. Wheat & rye

***NOTE** This is not an exhaustive list.*

The next step in treating SIBO or SIFO is to introduce what is called a "prokinetic."[115] A prokinetic encourages motility in the intestines, which will keep it clear so bacteria and fungus will not grow. Ginger root is a known natural prokinetic, but there are also prescription prokinetics.[116] Global Healing Center sells an excellent product called Oxy-Powder, which loosens compacted waste from the small intestine, large intestine, and colon. Oxy-Powder is an effective tool for combatting SIBO or SIFO. You can find it on their web site at: www.globalhealingcenter.com.

There are also many antibacterial and antifungal herbs that can help rid the intestines of an overgrowth of bad bugs, and I've listed some of the best ones below.

Antifungal Herbs to Combat SIFO:[117]

1. Turmeric
2. Pau d'arco
3. Olive leaf extract
4. Garlic
5. Black walnut
6. Tea tree (only use for limited time)
7. Cloves
8. Goldenseal
9. Oregano leaf oil
10. Calendula
11. Spearmint
12. Neem

Antibacterial Herbs to Combat SIBO:[118]

1. Grapefruit seed extract
2. Orgeno oil
3. Garlic
4. Berberine
5. Goldenseal
6. Olive leaf extract
7. Pau d'arco

Combination Herbs to Combat SIBO and SIFO:[119]

1. Dysbiocide by Biotics Research
2. FC-Cidal by Biotics Research
3. Biocidin by Bio-Batanical Research

4. Candibactin-AR & Candibactin-BR by Metagenics (taken together)

Before starting any herbal protocol, it is optimal to work with an experienced practitioner. Some of these herbs, whether taken alone or combined with other herbs, can be extremely potent. And some should only be taken for a short period of time. A naturopath or functional medicine practitioner experienced in working with herbs can help you determine which herbs are best for you and at what dosage. If you are struggling to find a practitioner near you, I've listed some recommended practitioners who are available via Skype consultation in Chapter 15.

Biofilm Busters: Enzymes & Herbs

Lyme disease, in particular, is hard to kill because it can shield itself in a biofilm (as can other infections), making it impenetrable to antibiotics.[120] It will therefore be important to supplement with "biofilm busters" while taking herbs targeted to kill infection. Some of these herbal protocols incorporate biofilm busters in their protocols, but some do not.

There are two main ways I approached biofilms, one was with enzymes and the other was with targeted herbs. Certain enzymes and herbs are effective at dissolving biofilm while also serving a dual purpose of aiding in various bodily functions. So, you are going to get a lot of bang for your buck using both enzymes and herbs together.

What Are Enzymes?

Enzymes are proteins the body uses to speed along chemical reactions inside cells.[121] From digestion, metabolism, repair and reproduction, we need enzymes for almost every bodily process.[122] The body creates enzymes on its own and we also ingest enzymes in the foods we eat. The more raw and fresh a food is, the more enzymes it will have. When we cook our food or process it, the enzymes are killed. One of the many problems with the standard American diet of overly processed and dead food is that it is lacking in enzymes. Add to this, we naturally produce fewer enzymes as we age.[123] There are two main types of enzymes, systemic and digestive, and they perform very important roles inside the body.

Systemic Enzymes

Systemic enzymes help to maintain our overall health. Specifically, they regulate inflammation and fibrin in the body.[124] This ability to break down fibrin is what makes them helpful in fighting infection, as biofilms that encapsulate infection are made up of fibrin.[125] Systemic enzymes can also help break down excess mucus, toxins, allergens, and clotting factors.[126] Generally speaking, systemic enzymes help keep all the body systems moving along smoothly.[127]

Digestive Enzymes

Digestive enzymes work in the gastrointestinal tract, helping the body to properly break down and digest fiber, protein, carbohydrates, and fats.[128] Issues such as bloating, indigestion, or gas are handled by our digestive enzymes or lack thereof.[129] If you suffer from any sort of digestive issues, such as gas, constipation, loose stools, indigestion, IBS, etc., you should consider taking a good quality digestive enzyme a few minutes before each meal. Even if you do not suffer obvious digestive distress, if you are chronically sick or have a weakened immune system, digestive enzymes may help ensure you absorb nutrients more efficiently from your food.

Benefits of Systemic Enzymes:[130]

1. Break down fibrin and helpful with fibrosis conditions (including biofilms and even ovarian cysts);

2. Break down scar tissue;
3. Improve circulation by breaking down cellular waste;
4. Improve white blood cell efficiency;
5. Can help manage overgrowth of yeast;
6. Help to manage inflammation within the body.

Benefits of Digestive Enzymes:[131]

1. Improve digestion and nutrient absorption by helping to break down food;
2. Alleviate dietary intolerances (relieves gas, bloating, and indigestion);
3. Support a proper microbiome balance.

My Favorite Biofilm Busters

1. **Cistus Incanus**
   Cistus incanus is an herb that can be taken as either a tea or tincture. I used this herb as a tea. Along with being able to break down biofilm, cistus is known to have antiviral, antibacterial, and antifungal properties.[132]

2. **Fars-P by Loomis Enzymes (Systemic Enzymes)**
   This systemic enzyme product worked incredibly well for me. It contains pancreatic enzymes, lipase, and calcium.[133] It is only available through licensed health-care practitioners, but often you can purchase such supplements after a simple and free phone consultation. This powerful enzyme supplement effectively ended my flu-like aches and pains within a week or two. Prior to starting with Fars-P, I had suffered with chronic flu-like body aches for close to two years. It was truly miraculous to me how well this product helped with inflammation and pain. How well it broke down biofilm is anyone's guess, but I can tell you my health improved by incorporating this enzyme formula.

3. **Serracor-NK by AST Enzymes & SerraRx by Biomedic Labs Rx (Systemic Enzymes)**

   These two systemic enzyme products continue to work incredibly well for me when taken together. Serracor-NK contains nattokinase, serrapeptase, bromelain, papain, lipase, proteases, rutin, amla, CoQ10, and magnesium.[134] SerraRx contains serrapeptase.[135] I quit using Fars-P after switching practitioners, and subsequently stumbled upon these products after considerable research on-line. I currently use them to curb pain from cysts and endometriosis. Cysts, just like biofilm, are made up of fibrin. And I can tell you, with the medical records to back it up, that these two products reduced the size of my cysts and have been incredible for easing pain. I fully trust they are equally effective at combatting biofilm simply because I know what they have done for my endometriosis symptoms. They are expensive, but I believe they work. While I take them together, you can also take them separately. I also admittedly take breaks from systemic enzymes and cannot vouch for using them routinely each day for more than five months or so at a time.

My Favorite Digestive Enzymes

1. **SpectraZyme by Metagest**

   This product contains betaine HCL and pepsin and should be taken with meals. Because it contains betaine hydrochloric acid, be sure you do not suffer stomach discomfort while taking it.

2. **Digestive Enzymes Ultra by Pure Encapsulations**

   This product has a nice variety of digestive enzymes, and like all digestive enzymes, should be taken with meals. Pure Encapsulations is a very well respected company by functional medicine practitioners. This product worked well for me and is reasonably priced.

There are many brands of digestive enzymes out there, so simply research and find what works best for you. These are my favorite products, but certainly there are lesser expensive options and products that may have a better formulation for your specific needs.

HCL For Heartburn & Acid Reflux

If you suffer heartburn or acid reflux, you may want to consider taking betaine hydrochloric acid (HCL) supplements as well.[136] What sometimes happens in cases of heartburn is the stomach stops producing enough acid (contrary to the popular belief that heartburn means *too much* acid!) to trigger the stomach door, so-to-speak, to close.[137] So, your food is churning in your stomach and acid splashes around and goes where it shouldn't—the esophagus.[138] By adding betaine HCL with your meals, you ensure that your stomach has the requisite amount of acid to trigger the stomach door to clamp tightly shut.[139] Working with a functional medicine practitioner can help you determine how much HCL you need to take. Generally speaking, I was told to take just enough so that I did not feel burning in my stomach after taking it. Once you take enough to feel burning, back down a tad bit.

Conclusion

There simply is no "magic bullet" of protocols to heal your body, and it is likely to take at least several different protocols for you to get well. But it is very important that you continually rotate a protocol into your regimen. If you aren't sure which protocol is best, just pick one and stick with it. Protocols such as Cowden's and Vital Plan are nice and easy because they take all the guess-work out of what to do, and provide a long term plan. If you know what infections you are battling, that is a major help, as obviously some herbs work better than others depending on specific infections. You can also devise your own protocols by buying individual herbs if you are motivated to do so. Stephen Buhner's books can give you a very good starting point from which to develop your own approach. For the most part, however, these herbal supplements are broad in range and will hit multiple infections at once. So, you may not need to pinpoint exactly what you're battling.

CHAPTER NINE

RECOVERY STEP #4— Restore Proper Balance to Your Microbiome

"If you think the pursuit of good health is expensive and time consuming, try illness."
Lee Swanson

Unfortunately, when we fall sick, it means we've likely damaged our gut microbiome such that beneficial bacteria may be either crowded out or killed off altogether.

Beneficial bacteria inside our bodies assist us in massive ways, from cancer prevention to mood regulation to the detoxification of toxins.[140] In a recent study at Cornell University, researchers demonstrated that CFS patients had less gut bacteria diversity, less anti-inflammatory bacteria, and more pro-inflammatory bacteria than their healthy counterparts.[141] In fact, as we've already discussed, researchers are also now learning that brain neurotransmitters, such as serotonin, are largely produced by the "good" bugs in our gut. Without question, the gut is command central for our immune system. It goes without saying that to get well, it is very important to repopulate the gut with beneficial bacteria.

There are several ways to properly re-inoculate the gut with beneficial bacteria, the first of which is to follow a healing diet, plentiful in leafy greens and low-sugar fruits and vegetables, as outlined herein. But, you should also consider supplementing with a high quality probiotic and prebiotic and adding a variety of fermented foods into your regimen.

Probiotics & Fermented Food

Probiotics are supplements that contain live and beneficial bacteria designed to repopulate the gut. Ideally, you are working with a decent functional medicine practitioner who will run tests to determine which probiotic supplement is best for you. I took a test at the Cleveland Clinic, for example, that identified bacteria I was deficient in so I could find a probiotic targeted to fit my needs.

There are numerous probiotic supplements to choose from. Generally speaking, however, you want to ensure you are not buying a cheap, two-strain probiotic supplement sold at your local drug store. The best quality probiotic supplements are going to be found at health food stores, typically in refrigerated cases, and will contain multiple strains of bacteria at a cost of at least $15-$20 or more per bottle.

There is much debate as to whether probiotic supplements can survive the acid in your stomach and therefore properly inoculate the gut. Some probiotics claim to be enteric coated and able to survive stomach acid and make it safely to the intestinal tract. It's anyone's guess if this does or does not happen. Regardless, I did rotate a good quality probiotic supplement that had at least ten or more strains for a good deal of my recovery period. As I progressed and was able to do more physically, however, I relied upon fermented food almost exclusively as my sole source of beneficial bacteria. Most high quality probiotics require refrigeration, although some do not. For this reason, be careful purchasing on-line over summer months as the hot temperatures can kill the bacteria in shipping.

If I had to recommend a single probiotic supplement, it would be MegaSporeBiotic. This product is unique in that it is a soil-based, spore-forming probiotic that adamantly professes to survive the acid of the stomach.[142] I've had several practitioners who do not sell this probiotic (and therefore have no "dog in the fight") sing its praises. This product also has a five year shelf-life, does not require refrigeration, and is alleged to maintain efficacy during antibiotic use.[143] Other good quality probiotic brands, in my opinion, include Renew Life, MegaFood, VSL #3 by The Living Shield, and Garden of Life.

As previously discussed in Chapter 6, you also want to introduce fermented foods, rich in beneficial bacteria, into your diet. Relying on expensive pills that may or may not work is not a sound plan. You will want to incorporate foods such as kefir, sauerkraut, kimchi, and kombucha on a regular basis. Fermented foods are easy and affordable to make at home, or you can find a decent variety in most grocery stores. Refer back to Chapter 6 for a more detailed discussion and tips on where to find great recipes.

Prebiotics

Prebiotics are essentially food for the "good" bugs in the gut. Specifically, prebiotics are non-digestible fiber compounds in food that pass through to the intestines where they stimulate the growth of beneficial bacteria.[144] Eating prebiotic rich foods and taking a prebiotic supplement can ensure your beneficial bacteria are thriving and multiplying. Examples of foods rich in prebiotics include onions, garlic, sweet potatoes, and bananas.[145] Prebiotic fiber powder can also be found in many health food stores. I routinely use a product by Hyperbiotics, aptly named "PreBiotic."

It contains an organic prebiotic fiber blend that includes acacia fiber, Jerusalem artichoke fiber, and zuvii green banana flour.

Pumping the Breaks on Fermented Food: SIBO & SIFO

There are some situations in which fermented foods may exacerbate your problems. It is believed that some people do not respond well to D-lactate, which is an acid produced by some probiotic bacteria, including Lactobacillus acidophilus.[146] If you are one of these people, it is recommended that you instead opt for a probiotic containing strains of Bifidobacterium.[147] Also, if you've been diagnosed with small intestinal bacterial overgrowth (SIBO) or small intestinal fungal overgrowth (SIFO), you will likely have a difficult time adding fermented foods into your diet. As previously discussed, if you suffer from SIBO or SIFO, it means that food is sitting partially undigested in your small intestine creating bacteria and dysbiosis. Eating bacteria-rich fermented food would add gas to the fire.

Conclusion

Repopulating the gut with beneficial bacteria is a critical step to healing, and while time-consuming, it is not difficult to accomplish. It simply requires you to commit to a diet that promotes the growth of beneficial microbe strains. By consistently choosing low-sugar fruits, incorporating plenty of green leafy vegetables, fermented foods, probiotics, and prebiotic foods or supplements, you will make slow and steady gains. This is not a one-month or six-month plan. This is a lifestyle. Before you eat a meal, ask yourself if it is what your gut needs to heal. If it isn't, then you are likely contributing to a disease state. It's that simple. The better choices you make at each and every meal, the better you will feel over time. You will make mistakes, and you will have days where you crash and eat the cookie. But don't make that a habit. Always pick yourself back up and get back at it. Like Babe Ruth said, "[i]t's hard to beat a person who never gives up."

CHAPTER TEN

RECOVERY STEP #5— Implement Gentle Detox & Support Modalities

"If we are facing in the right direction, all we have to do is keep on walking."
Zen Proverb

Throughout this process of cleaning up your gut, you will need to support your body's natural detoxification processes. You may notice that as you add in an herbal protocol, you begin to feel more sick. As discussed briefly in Chapter 1, this is because the infection(s) is dying faster than your body can detoxify it. The dead waste can build up, especially in a person with a compromised immune system, resulting in what is called a "Jarisch-Herxheimer Reaction," or "Herxheimer" or "herx" for short.[148] If you are like me, you are a slow metabolizer and a slow "detoxer." Always listen to your body, and if you feel particularly wiped out, back off from all of your supplements and give your body a rest. Do not go faster than your body can comfortably tolerate. Regaining your health is not a sprint, it's a long process. Be patient and kind to yourself.

Also, be leery of products marketed to detoxify your body. Your body was created to detoxify itself. Your job is simply to *support* the detoxification process. You do not need to spend a lot of money on fancy supplements or complex detox programs in order to detox. Your liver knows how to do its job, it just needs you to support it by eating a clean diet and taking care of your body.

My Favorite Detoxification Support

1. **Filtered Water**

    Drink lots of clean, filtered water throughout the day, sometimes with freshly squeezed lemon. Lemon is excellent for your liver, which is the critical organ in detoxification. The water filter I use is Zero Water, and I highly recommend it. However, I've had practitioners also recommend the Big Berkey water filtration system. Whichever filtration system you choose, just be sure it works! Clean water is important.

2. **Herbal Tea**

    Drink herbal tea, particularly dandelion root. Dandelion root is believed to help increase the flow of bile, and therefore help detoxify the liver.

3. **Oxy-Powder by Global Healing Center**

    This product is helpful as an intestinal cleanse or to relieve occasional constipation. It is said to literally melt away compaction from the small intestine, large intestine, and colon. This is not a supplement to stay on long term, but to perform periodic intestinal cleansing. I have used it several times and found it helpful, especially when combatting SIBO or SIFO.

4. **Gemmotherapies**

    Gemmotherapies use the fresh buds and young shoots of developing plants to treat a variety of ailments and conditions.

I found them helpful with detoxification. But, they can also be used in a myriad of ways to treat various conditions under the care of a licensed naturopath. They can be potent and take training to truly understand, so it is best to work with a trained practitioner to properly implement them. In Chapter 15, I provide contact information for a naturopath (Jennifer Sierzant) who is very proficient in the use of these remedies.

5. **Diatomaceous Earth ("DE")**

    DE, as discussed in the previous chapter, is made up of the fossilized remains of diatoms, which are a type of algae found in river and lake beds.[149] The cell walls of these diatoms are made of silica and they easily break down into a fine powder. DE is said to kill parasites and viruses while cleaning the digestive tract, improving liver function, and absorbing harmful chemicals in the blood.[150] You must be sure that your DE is **food grade**, however, before ingesting. It is easy to take, simply add a teaspoon to a tablespoon in water and drink once daily. As an aside, I used DE for a limited duration, so please discuss with your practitioner if you plan to use it daily for more than a month or so.

6. **Exercise**

    No matter how light and minimal, exercise helps get the lymphatic system moving, blood flowing, and simply helps the body in all areas. The more you can move, the better you are going to feel. No matter your situation, do what you can. Even if you cannot break a sweat, you can improve your circulation with something as simple as stretching, and that is important to clear the body of toxins. Please see Chapter 11 for a detailed discussion on the many benefits of exercise.

7. **Sauna**

    If tolerable, saunas are an excellent detox modality. I used a Richway Amethyst Biomat at my sickest, as I could simply lay on the infrared heated mat while it warmed my body, helping me work up a light sweat. The Biomat is an electric mat containing crystals that release infrared heat into the body. You can research this mat at:

    https://www.healingartsgarden.com/product/biomat-professional-7000mx-74x28

    I've also used portable infrared saunas, which can be purchased relatively cheaply on Amazon for around $200. Your local gym may have a sauna of some variety as well. Working up a sweat, though, can be taxing when you are in the throes of a chronic illness, so be very careful and go slowly. You don't want to over-do it.

8. **Sleep**

    Most importantly, get plenty of sleep! Sleep allows your brain to regroup, repair, and remove toxic waste byproducts that have accumulated throughout the day. One of those waste products is called beta-amyloid, which contributes to the development of Alzheimer's disease.[151] Sleep is critical, so make sure it is a major focus and a priority.

General Support – Multivitamins

Supporting your body with a high quality multivitamin may also be necessary while you are acutely sick. Working with a functional medicine practitioner will be beneficial here, as he or she can perform bloodwork to determine if you are lacking in certain vitamins or minerals. If you are following *The Wahls Protocol*, she encourages you to focus on food as your primary source of vitamins. So at some point, you will want to scale back on your reliance on supplements and focus more on your diet. However, there are situations where a multivitamin is beneficial. I did take a few multivitamins while sick, and I've listed my favorite ones below.

My Favorite Multivitamins

1. **PureGenomics Multivitamin by Pure Encapsulations**
   This supplement is an excellent one-a-day vitamin tailored for people who have genetic variations in their methylation pathways. In simple terms, this means it is for people who have a hard time absorbing vitamins. Often times people with chronic conditions have genetic mutations, such as MTHFR, mentioned earlier, that prevent them from properly metabolizing certain vitamins. Pure Encapsulations is a well trusted, high quality vitamin brand.

2. **Prevention Plus by Vital Plan**
   This supplement contains a mixture of herbs, vitamins and minerals. It also contains activated B vitamins to ensure proper absorption. As previously discussed, some people do not absorb B vitamins properly unless they are in a methylated form.

3. **Mega Food Vitamins**
   Mega Food multivitamins are made from real food, which is the optimal source of any vitamin or mineral. They have a wide range of vitamins based upon your specific needs. You can find all of their supplements at: www.megafood.com.

Conclusion

Supporting your body throughout the healing process is very important. Take extra measures to be loving and patient with yourself. Your body needs time and space to heal. Ensure it gets this by supporting it in every way possible. Sticking to your nutrient-dense diet, getting plenty of water, sleeping regularly, and implementing the detoxification support methods outlined above will help to streamline your recovery.

And remember—the path to success and well-being is not linear. It is marked with many peaks and many deep valleys. As you start to feel a bit better, oddly the valleys feel much worse. It's because, as you find yourself getting a taste of feeling better, falling backward is just all the more devastating. Know in those times that your setback is only temporary and a normal part of the recovery process. Over time, your worst days will start to be much less severe. One day, you will realize that your worst days are what your best days used to be. Stick to the guidelines I've outlined, and work with a trained practitioner if possible to tweak your protocol along the way. You can do it!

CHAPTER ELEVEN

RECOVERY STEP #6— Restore Energy with Targeted Nutrition, Exercise, and Supplementation

"Restore your soul. Replenish your energy. Seek yourself. No matter whether you have been pushed or pulled by situations and people, it has only lead to one thing – growth."
Nishtha Grover

R egaining my energy has been the biggest battle in my fight against Lyme disease and chronic illness. After years of dealing with a long litany of torturous symptoms, I found myself *almost* well except for one small thing—my energy was gone. My daily flu-like aches had subsided, my body tremors were ancient history, no more random stabbing pains in my legs and joints, and I no longer suffered severe brain fog, or recurrent weakness on the entire right side of my body. I'd found a way to reduce or completely reverse nearly every single symptom, but reversing my fatigue was, and continues to be, my biggest hurdle.

While I am not back to running marathons, I have very significantly improved my energy, to a point where I can offer legitimate and insightful wisdom on the topic. A few short years ago, I lacked the energy to walk to my mailbox and back without feeling unstable and needing to rest. Now, I am jogging about two miles several times per week, or at a minimum speed-walking 1.5 miles. I then try to finish my workout with weight training for 15 to 20 minutes. If the weather does not permit me a jog or walk, I swim for 30 minutes and weight train afterward. Most significantly, I suffer very little post-exertion malaise now after completing a workout. Whereas before, after completing any sort of physical exertion, I would end up relegated to the bed or the sofa for hours or days.

Granted, these workouts are a far cry from the daily four mile runs I completed with ease prior to falling sick. But, these workouts represent a very significant improvement in my energy levels, and for that I am grateful. Not only am I now completing these workouts regularly, but I also have the stamina to get through a normal day with two active children. By following the principles I've outlined in this book, my energy continues to improve week over week, month over month, and year over year. At this stage, I expect to fully restore my energy in the months ahead.

I want to emphasize that I am still a work in progress, and I still have days where I fall apart and must lay down mid-day. I still have days where I must take things more slowly, demonstrate patience with myself, and listen to my body. And these are all things that you must also do to get well and restore your energy. **You will not improve your energy by pushing yourself too quickly.** Meet yourself wherever you are and work from there!

Four Key Steps to Restoring Your Energy

In my experience, there are four keys to restoring your energy both during and following chronic illness, and they are as follows:

(1) Strict adherence to a nutrient-dense diet, devoid of processed foods, sugar, starchy carbs, and any foods that specifically cause *you* sensitivity;

(2) Restorative sleep;

(3) Properly tailored exercise; and

(4) Properly tailored supplementation.

The first three items in this list are of critical importance. The last item, supplementation, may help you achieve quicker results, but it may also do absolutely nothing. Your focus should be on items 1-3, adding only the supplementation that you feel is helpful. I have already spoken at length on the proper diet required to restore your health and therefore your energy, so we will move directly to restorative sleep.

Slaying the Sleep Dragon – Beating Insomnia & Achieving Restorative Sleep

Emil Cioran, a Romanian philosopher, once aptly noted that, "[i]nsomnia is a vertiginous lucidity that can convert paradise itself into a place of torture."

I almost hate to broach the topic of insomnia for fear I will awaken the beast, and it will return. Of all the symptoms I have suffered, insomnia might be the most torturous. And sadly, I'm not sure one can escape Lyme disease or any severe chronic illness without suffering from it. It can become a literal bear on your back, convincing you that death is imminent. But, the fact remains that sleep is critical to recovery, and insomnia must be tackled.

My insomnia became so persistent and intolerable that I resorted to pharmaceutical drugs for help. That was a major mistake, in hindsight. I'd gone so many nights without sleep, however, I felt it was an emergency and just took the pills. The first prescription I tried was Ambien. It certainly worked for the first few days. But over time, it completely stopped working, and my insomnia became a thousand percent worse. I became completely incapable of shutting my brain down for sleep. No matter how tired I was, I'd lay in my bed in sheer agony unable to get any amount of sleep. So, I increased my dose of Ambien, which helped some nights, but mostly just exacerbated my problem.

Over time, I realized that not only was the sleep medication not working, but it was making my insomnia much more severe and giving me significant memory problems as well. I had to stop.

Quitting Ambien was not easy. In fact, it was so difficult that I ended up back at the doctor's office pleading for some other alternative sleep medication. I was given another medication (I cannot remember its name), and it made my eyes feel so heavy I could barely see straight. The next morning after taking it, I felt like someone had clobbered me with a baseball bat. It was only then that I resolved to regain my ability to sleep without the help of medication, no matter how difficult.

My best advice to anyone battling severe insomnia is not to panic. Even if you find yourself unable to sleep, try to simply roll with it. Don't freak out – like I did! It is very hard when you're on night three or four with no sleep, already extremely exhausted from fighting an illness, and the sleep you need desperately just won't happen. But the more you fight the current, the more the current will wear you down. Just go with the flow. The next day might be difficult, but you will get through it. So try to relax.

Sleep hygiene is critical. Be sure that as night-time approaches, you are slowly but surely getting ready for sleep. Lower the lights. Turn off your cell phone and tablet. Do not eat a big meal within the few hours before bed. Ensure that your bedroom is conducive to sleeping. This may mean running a fan for "white noise," putting up black-out curtains to block ambient light from outside, and shutting off your television if you have one in your bedroom. Also, taking a warm shower before bed is an excellent idea, as it naturally relaxes your body for better sleep.

Exercise is the next very crucial step to a good night of sleep, and I will discuss in more depth in the next section. If you've been sick for any period of time, you will understand what I mean by feeling tired but wired. You want to sleep, but feel like you have electricity running through your veins. Exercise will help alleviate this feeling and make it easier for your brain to shift into a calm state for sleep. It will relax your muscles, improve blood flow, and help your body to balance its hormones. With consistent exercise, you will once again feel truly ready to fall asleep at night with little effort.

Obviously, exercise is not so easy when you are sick. It is difficult to get your body moving—maybe nearly impossible. But the body was not meant to lay around all day, no matter how poorly you feel. During the day, try to lift light weights, or stretch—anything to get your blood flowing. I forced myself to get back into the pool and do light exercises while going through the worst of my insomnia, and this was a critical step in restoring my sleep. The resistance work felt great on my muscles, and it had a relaxing effect on me at night. Initially, I was not swimming laps, but merely doing some resistance work in the water and swimming short widths of the pool. Simply do what you are capable of doing. You may surprise yourself and find you are able to do more than you thought you could.

Not being able to sleep is a real physical problem. It means your sleep hormones are out of whack, and you likely have high cortisol levels at night. My functional medicine practitioner ran a test on me that demonstrated precisely why I was not sleeping. My hormones were flip flopped. My cortisol was sky high at night when it was supposed to be low to induce sleep. Then, in the morning, when cortisol should rise to wake me up, it was too low. These hormone imbalances take time and patience to correct, but they can be worked out naturally without the harmful side effects of pharmaceutical drugs.

If cortisol is a problem for you, there are supplements that can specifically work to help restore proper cortisol levels. Ashwagandha has been shown to lower cortisol levels if they are too high, and it is what I used to restore my hormone balance. As previously discussed, it is an adaptogenic herb, meaning it aids the body's stress response by helping to balance cortisol during the day. I would take my first dose around dinner time when my tests showed my cortisol levels would start to rise. I would take my second dose at bed time. Cortisol Manager by Integrative Therapeutics is also often recommended by functional medicine practitioners, although I did not take this particular product. I have read numerous positive reviews for it and would certainly try it if ashwaghanda did not provide relief.

Below are the sleep supplements I used at bedtime along with ashwagandha to gradually restore my sleep. Of course, I did not use them all at once. I used different ones at different times, as I would find that one might work for a while and then stop working so well. It is a matter of trial and error determining what works for *you*. Natural Calm can always be taken with any of the other supplements, as it is essentially a magnesium supplement. I would also often combine Gaia Herb's Sleep Thru supplement with Best Rest with a very good result.

My Recommended Sleep Supplements:

1. Best Rest by Pure Encapsulations
2. Sleep Thru by Gaia Herbs

3. Sound Sleep by Gaia Herbs
4. Ashwagandha by Pure Encapsulations
5. Holy Basil
6. L-Theanine
7. Kavinace
8. PheniTropic
9. Natural Calm Plus Calcium by Natural Vitality

I still have nights and short stretches, like any human being, where I struggle with sleep. But for the most part, I now get a full eight hours of sleep *every* night. I suffered with severe insomnia for the better part of two years. It was absolute and pure hell. If you are going through it right now, follow the steps I've outlined religiously, figure out what supplements work for you, and go easy on yourself. On nights when you cannot fall asleep, remember to stay calm. I would often get up and do sit-ups or push-ups on the side of my bed to shake out my muscles. The wired but tired feeling is not pleasant, but it will get better.

And always remember, insomnia is just one more bump in the road on your way to wellness. Your sleep will improve over time.

Exercise Massively Improves Energy

Being chronically sick and immobile for a long period of time can radically damage your mitochondria, the powerhouses of your cells.[152] Fortunately, exercise can help repair and protect the damage done to your mitochondria and restore your energy levels.[153]

Each and every time you exercise, you create more mitochondria. I repeat: ***each and every time you exercise, you create more mitochondria***. Your body was made to move, period, and exercise will be a critical component to your healing. As one of my practitioners succinctly put it to me, "*if you want to lose weight, focus on diet. But if you want to restore or improve your energy, you must exercise.*" While I was not interested in losing weight, I became acutely aware each time I exercised that my energy was improving. He was absolutely correct and my body was confirming it.

In addition to impacting energy production, exercise also improves your balance, flexibility, muscle tone, circulation, and maybe most importantly, your mood.[154] When you exercise, your body produces endorphins, which are chemicals in the brain that give you a sense of well-being and help reduce pain.[155] You know that euphoric and relaxed feeling that washes over you after a walk or run? Thank your endorphins.

Exercise is the proverbial miracle pill. It can do incredible things on many levels for your body. But how do you exercise if you can barely get out of bed?

Whatever Exercise You Can Do – DO IT!

My advice is to meet yourself wherever you are. Don't try to do anything you simply cannot do. But, even if you are bedridden, you can likely do light stretching, maybe leg lifts, use resistance bands, and possibly even lift light hand-weights. Do whatever it is you are capable of doing. The goal is to get the muscles moving and improve blood flow, not necessarily to get your heartrate elevated or break a sweat.

In the beginning, I found that any sort of aerobic exercise absolutely decimated me. A walk to the mailbox was a marathon for my body. I had no stamina or ability to replenish energy. Any time I tried to do anything that required any sort of exertion, I would get pushed back and paid the price for about a week. Resistance exercises, however, were another story. Sit-ups, push-ups, and lifting light hand-weights actually gave me a bit of an energy boost without totally wiping me out. I never got myself completely out of breath, but I got my muscles working again.

Initially, you will want to proceed very slowly to see how you respond to exercise. When you're chronically sick, your body is fragile. You can cross the line and do too much very easily without knowing it. My very light workout with hand-weights slowly graduated to climbing my stairs repeatedly, and then to swimming two to three times per week at the gym. Returning to the gym was a *huge* milestone for me. I was very gentle on myself, however, and started with swimming just the width of the pool for about five minutes at a time. After a few months, my stamina improved such that I was able to swim lengths of the pool.

Still some weeks, I couldn't swim at all. And that was fine. Always listen to your body and don't beat yourself up. You will have days and weeks where you just can't do anything. Rest assured that this is all part of the healing process. As discussed previously, the path to success is **NOT** linear!!! But as you keep up with your diet, herbal protocols, and proper sleep hygiene, you will find yourself generally able to do more and more every day.

Eventually, I was also able to go for walks. Going on walks was something I had avoided altogether in the mid-stages of my recovery because walking depleted my energy. Over time, though, as my stamina improved, I found that walking did not wear me out as much. Instead, I found it to be incredibly invigorating and therapeutic. Being outdoors is so beneficial for your body and spirit, so if you can tolerate a walk, I recommend it. Breathing deeply as you walk, being present mentally, being grateful for your life and family, and simply noticing the trees, birds, and sky is incredibly cathartic. Walking for me was a form of meditation that helped me feel like a human being again. I did not walk far at first, just a few blocks from my house and back.

Just as with swimming, the walks slowly increased in pace and duration until one day I almost broke down in tears realizing I'd walked an entire mile at a fairly brisk pace. For someone who'd spent two years in bed and her disability money on a burial plot, this was an amazing feeling. I'm now very proud to report I can jog that distance and more!

The "I'm Too Tired" Cycle

The problem you will face is that you don't *feel* like exercising. It's completely warranted and understandable, and I had the same problem. You feel *so extremely* tired that you must lay down a lot, which then leads to you feeling even more tired. But it becomes a vicious cycle that you must break. Just because you feel like lying down doesn't always mean you should.

It's a tightrope walk, without question, and you do not want to do more than your body can tolerate. But, you also do not want to do far less. Take your time, listen to your body, and keep things simple. *But do exercise, nonetheless.* I cannot tell you how many days I waddled into the gym walking slower than the old ladies with walkers on their way to their "Golden Ladies Water Aerobics Class." On most days headed into the gym, I truly felt that I could very well be taken out in an ambulance. But, I did it anyway. I'd take it one stroke, or lap, at a time and see how I felt, always pushing myself to do as much as I could without over-doing. And to my surprise, I almost always felt better after my swim. My brain fog improved, my energy perked up, my muscles felt relaxed and more toned. I'd also find I was able to get through the dinner hour at home with my kids with stamina I'd otherwise not have had.

As discussed earlier, exercise also helped dramatically improve my sleep, which in turn, improved my energy. If you suffer from insomnia, exercise is an important key to restoring your circadian rhythm. Your body was made to move and to become tired naturally from a day of physical activity. When you are cooped up all day in bed or limiting your movement, everything gets thrown out of balance. Your hormones aren't being produced as they should, your muscles atrophy, your circulation becomes sluggish, and as a result your sleep pattern gets disrupted. If you've been sick and immobile for a significant period, all the more reason you must begin to exercise again.

Please remember to go easy on yourself, listen to your body, and celebrate with each workout how far you've come. There will still be days, maybe even extended periods, where your energy once again plummets and you find yourself unable to do much. Honor your body during these times and what it's telling you. Don't beat yourself up. You will eventually rebound and get back at it. This cycling of good and bad periods is what recovery looks like, no matter how frustrating that may feel. But making exercise a regular part of your week—when and if you are capable of doing so—may be the missing piece to your recovery.

Targeted Supplementation

There are endless supplements marketed to boost energy, but many of them are total bogus. If you are not eating properly and following a diet such as *The Wahls Protocol*, do not even bother with energy supplements. Food is your medicine, and supplements should be just that—*supplemental* to your already nutrient-dense diet and properly tailored exercise regimen. With this said, there are a few worthwhile supplements targeted to help struggling mitochondria and energy production, and I've listed below the ones I feel might provide the most promise.

1. **D-Ribose**

    D-ribose is a simple sugar and an essential component to adenosine triphosphate (ATP), which is necessary for cellular energy.[156] The body creates d-ribose naturally, but many practitioners recommend d-ribose in supplemental form for those suffering with chronic fatigue syndrome or fibromyalgia, although there are few studies on its efficacy. A small study in The Journal of Alternative and Complementary Medicine concluded that it significantly improved energy levels, sleep quality, mental clarity, pain intensity, and overall well-being.[157] It's also been shown to increase exercise capacity and energy following a heart attack.[158] The only true way to know if it can give you any sort of benefit is to try it. The recommended dosage is anywhere from 5 grams once daily to 15 grams daily in three divided doses. I can say with a fair degree of certainty that d-ribose has helped restore my energy, and I continue to use it to this day.

2. Acetyl-L-Carnitine & Alpha Lipoic Acid

These two supplements taken together are purported to improve cognitive functioning and mental energy. According to researchers, alpha lipoic acid is the strongest antioxidant rejuvenator of aging brains ever seen in aged animals, and it's especially powerful if combined with acetyl-l-carnitine.[159] In one study, old and sluggish rats given daily doses of both supplements became as physically and mentally active as rats half their age within weeks.[160] In explaining these results, researchers noted that acetyl-l-carnitine works as fuel to keep mitochondria working well. As we age, we create less and less acetyl-l-carnitine, so supplementation seems an appropriate approach. Alpha lipoic acid aids brain cells in protecting mitochondria from damage.[161] Alpha lipoic acid is considered safe at 200 mg per day, and acetyl-l-carnitine is recommended at 500 mg per day.[162]

3. NAC

N-acetyl cysteine is a supplement form of cysteine. Cysteine is a semi-essential amino acid, which becomes essential if dietary intake of methionine and serine is low.[163] Cysteine is found in high-protein foods such as chicken, turkey, eggs, and legumes. NAC is needed along with glutamine and glycine to create glutathione.[164] Glutathione recycles antioxidants in the body, helps our immune system fight infection and prevent cancer, aids in detoxification, and aids the body in physical and mental function by decreasing muscle damage, reducing recovery time, and helping increase strength and endurance.[165] Because of NAC's critical role in the production of glutathione, it is often recommended in supplement form to ensure optimal glutathione levels. Although, it is worth noting that NAC is not very well absorbed by the body, so your best bet may be to stick to food sources of cysteine. The accepted daily recommended dose of NAC is 600 – 1800 mg.[166]

4. **Magnesium**

   Magnesium is one of my favorite supplements. It's estimated that 50% of the population is deficient in this mineral, which is found abundantly in dark leafy greens, nuts, avocados, and dark chocolate.[167] Magnesium is known to activate adenosine triphosphate or "ATP" in the body, which in turn helps to create energy.[168] It is also highly regarded for its anti-inflammatory effects and its ability to help regulate neurotransmitters in the brain.[169] The daily recommended dose for magnesium is about 400 mg per day.

5. **CoQ10**

   CoQ10 helps to generate energy in your cells and low levels have been linked to conditions such as heart disease, brain disorders, diabetes and cancer. With age, naturally occurring levels of CoQ10 decrease.[170] Foods containing CoQ10 include organ meats, chicken, beef, fatty fish, spinach, and broccoli.[171] When supplementing, there are two forms of CoQ10 to consider: Ubiquinone and Ubiquinol. When Ubiquinone is used by the body, it must be converted to Ubiquinol. Ubiquinone is the conventional oxidized form of CoQ10, and can be difficult for the body to convert.[172] So, it stands to reason that the Ubiquinol form might be better absorbed by the body, as it is already broken down into the active form of CoQ10. Generally speaking, a reasonable daily dose of CoQ10 is 100 – 300 mg, although it has been shown to be safe up to 1200 mg.[173]

6. B Complex Vitamin

B vitamins help convert food into glucose, and hence give you energy. Specifically, vitamin B12 helps to keep your nerves and blood cells healthy and guards against pernicious anemia, which can make you feel very tired.[174] It is estimated that 10-30% of adults do not properly absorb vitamin B12 from the food they eat, while many others simply fail to follow a proper diet and are accordingly low in B vitamins.[175] I recommend Pure Encapsulations B-Complex Plus, as it has the proper methylated and absorbable form of B vitamins, and it comes highly regarded by most practitioners.

There are, of course, other herbs and supplements that may help boost energy production. One other supplement worth mentioning is creatine monohydrate. Creatine may help curb post-exertion malaise and improve blood flow and oxidative stress.[176] I admittedly shied away from most products specifically marketed to increase energy, because they tend to give me negative side effects in the form of insomnia and heart palpitations. I also don't buy into the marketing hype of many of these products. Also worth noting, an iron deficiency, thyroid, or genetic condition could be the cause of your fatigue, each of which would require blood work to diagnose and properly treat.

Conclusion

Fatigue can have so many different causes, it is a difficult symptom to tackle. First and foremost, it is important to have a thorough medical examination with bloodwork to rule out genetic disorders or other known and treatable diseases. That said, by taking a wide approach and (1) ensuring your diet is nourishing your cells and mitochondria, (2) giving your body the proper time to recover by sleeping 7-8 hours per night, (3) consistently implementing an appropriate exercise routine, and (4) adding targeted supplementation to give your body an extra boost, you are likely to see your energy levels improve. It will not happen overnight. Remember, this is a war of attrition – you must stick to the program for the long haul. But over time, you should certainly feel your energy level start to budge. That success will beget more success, until one day you have to pinch yourself because you have stamina to do things you haven't done in years!

CHAPTER TWELVE

RECOVERY STEP #7— Detoxify Your Environment

"Be as simple as you can be; you will be astonished to see how uncomplicated and happy your life can become."
Paramahansa Yogonanda

Take a good hard look at all of the toxic exposure your body endures over the course of a single day. From electromagnetic field (EMF) radiation, to the chemicals in your shampoo, soaps, body lotions, makeup, cleaning products, air conditioning systems, environmental pollutants—especially if you live in a densely populated city, and the endless chemicals and toxic substances in our processed food and tap water, your body is absolutely bombarded with toxins taxing it unnecessarily. And when you are fighting a disease, your body simply cannot handle an attack on all fronts. Starting today, you need to do everything you can to limit your exposure to unnecessary toxic burdens.

Drinking Water

Let's first examine drinking water. Remember, you don't just drink water, you breathe it as steam when you shower and absorb it through your skin. In 2008, it was reported that a "vast array" of pharmaceutical drugs including sex hormones, mood stabilizers, antibiotics, ibuprofen, acetaminophen, and heart and cholesterol drugs were found in the drinking water of 24 major US cities impacting at least 41 million Americans.[177] Anti-epileptic and anti-anxiety medications were found in the drinking water in southern California impacting 18.5 million.[178] And the drinking water in our nation's capital, of all places, tested positive for six different pharmaceutical drugs.[179] Think you might want to start filtering your water? That answer is a definite YES.

There are two water filtration systems I recommend. One is Zero Water, and the other is Berkey. I have been using Zero Water for many years now, and I love it. Zero Water offers the largest refrigerator dispenser of any other filtration system, which is a huge selling feature for me.[180] If you like your water cold and you drink a lot of it, this system may be perfect for you. Other systems with large capacity dispensers cannot fit inside a refrigerator and instead take up prime real estate on your countertop. According to Zero Water's web site, its filtration system removes 99.9% of all detectable solids.[181] Detectable solids are non-organic impurities that come from rusty pipes, run-off from road salt, pesticides, fertilizers and more. Zero Water has been independently tested to reduce fluoride by up to 99%, as well as pharmaceutical drugs, arsenic, lead, and chloramine.[182] For an exhaustive list of everything this filter is effective against, visit the Zero Water web site at www.zerowater.com. Their filtration system is quite affordable, at about $40 for a 30 cup dispenser plus the cost of filters. Filters cost about $15 each and will need to be replaced about every four weeks or so, dependent upon how much water you drink.

The Berkey water filtration system has been recommended to me several times by various practitioners. But, due to its cost and having never felt the need to abandon Zero Water, I've yet to personally try it. I recommend it because I trust the people who have repeatedly vouched for it. Berkey contends that its filters are more powerful than any other gravity filter currently available.[183] Each Berkey system will last for up to 3000 gallons of water, or 6000 gallons per set, and can remove (to greater than 99.9%) fluoride, viruses, pathogenic bacteria, lead, arsenic, iron, mercury, chlorine, chloramines, pesticides, and pharmaceuticals to greater than 99.5%.[184] This is not an exhaustive list, so visit their web site at www.berkeyfilters.com for more information. A Big Berkey system holds 2.25 gallons of water and costs about $300, plus the cost of filters which run around $125 for a set of two.[185] So, while this is a large financial investment, it is a high quality water filtration system.

Berkey also offers shower head filters, which are obviously a great idea for anyone who is immune compromised. As mentioned earlier, you don't just drink your water, you bathe in it. If you don't want to drink what's coming out of your tap, you probably don't want to shower in it either. Their shower filters sell for about $70 and last for about 25,000 gallons of water or one year, whichever comes first.[186]

There are of course other companies out there that offer water filtration systems for your home and shower. Do your research and select the product and company you feel most comfortable with. But do not assume that any filtration system out there will "do." As an example, Brita sells a popular filtration system, but in my experience, it does not even compare to others such as Zero Water and Berkey.

Anything Applied to Your Skin

Lotions, soaps, fragrances, cosmetics, laundry detergents and dryer sheets all contain toxic chemicals that may enter your body through your skin. This is not to say that anything applied to the skin enters the bloodstream, as some chemicals are molecularly too large. But, some chemicals can and do. Take for instance, prescription hormone creams or prescription skin patches for nicotine addiction and pain management. These drugs work by entering the blood stream via the skin. You are wise to give pause to any product you use daily on your body and skin to ensure its ingredients are safe.

1. **Parabens, Fluoride, & Heavy Metals**

    Parabens are synthetic preservatives meant to prevent the growth of fungus and bacteria in products such as toothpaste, deodorant, shampoo, cosmetics, and body lotion.[187] If the product you use contains methylparaben, ethylparaben, propylparaben, butylparaben, or isobutylparaben, then it has parabens.[188] Researchers have also found that approximately 90% of common grocery items contain a measurable amount of parabens.[189] This means parabens are insidious in both our food and body products and are therefore difficult to avoid altogether.

    Parabens are known hormone disruptors, and are linked to increased breast cancer and reproductive problems.[190] It is believed that parabens may interact with growth factors in the body to increase the risk of breast cancer.[191] In a study conducted at UC Berkley, researchers discovered that parabens triggered estrogen receptors by turning on genes that caused the cells to significantly proliferate.[192] The UC Berkley study also suggests that the potential negative effects of parabens at lower doses may have been underestimated, and that current safety testing for parabens may not accurately predict their impact upon human health.[193]

    Also worth noting, products such as toothpaste and mouthwash may not only contain parabens but also fluoride. While too little fluoride is linked to cavities and tooth decay, there are also health risks associated with too much exposure.[194] In 2014, The Lancet medical journal designated fluoride as a neurotoxin, which led US officials to lower fluoride levels in drinking water for the first time in 50 years.[195] While the debate on fluoride's benefits and dangers lingers on, it's probably best to err on the side of caution. A diet low in sugar along with sound dental hygiene, which includes flossing and brushing three times per day, should keep your teeth in good shape without the use of fluoride.[196]

Everyday heavy metal exposure may also contribute to chronic health problems. Many deodorants, for example, contain aluminum, a heavy metal linked to Alzheimer's, ALS, and autism.[197] Aluminum foil wrap may also pose a potential risk, especially if used under high heat when cooking. Mercury fillings in your teeth are believed by some dental experts to be toxic to the body. Some dentists contend that the mercury—a known neurotoxin—can leach into the body.[198] There are dentists who specialize in the proper removal of mercury fillings if you suspect you have such a problem.

Simply make your best effort to avoid using potentially toxic products on or near your body. There are many companies out there that cater to health-conscious consumers and use safe ingredients in their personal hygiene products.

2. Chemicals in Dryer Sheets

Dryer sheets are a common product many people overlook as a source of toxins. However, the chemicals and fragrances in these sheets can mimic estrogen in the body and also contribute to asthma and allergy symptoms.[199] Sadly, you do not even know what you are rubbing on your skin while wearing clothing dried with a dryer sheet. The US Consumer Product Safety Commission does not require manufacturers to list the chemical ingredients in their dryer sheets.[200] You may love that faux flowery smell, but know that with that fragrance comes a smorgasbord of chemicals.

According to EcoWatch, dryer sheets often contain quaternary ammonium compounds and can routinely trigger reproductive toxicity in animals.[201] While testing every day household products for hormone disruptors and asthma triggers, the Silent Spring Institute researchers found dryer sheets to contain some of the highest amounts of toxic fragrance chemicals, as well as acetyl hexamethyl tetralin, isobornyl acetate and phenethyl alcohol.[202] In other studies, researchers reported that 44% of scented laundry products tested contained at least one carcinogenic hazardous air pollutant, to include acetaldehyde, 1,4-dioxane, and formaldehyde.[203] Some common side effects from inhaling dryer vent emissions when dyer sheets were used include asthma attacks, respiratory problems, runny nose, migraines, gastrointestinal distress, and skin irritation.[204]

Do your best to find plant-based, fragrance-free laundry detergents and avoid dryer sheets altogether. To avoid static with your laundry, Dr. Axe recommends a quarter cup of white vinegar added to your rinse cycle or conversely to use a wool dryer ball.[205]

3. **Chemicals in Clothing**

If you're like me, you also never thought about clothing as a source of toxic chemicals. In fact, it wasn't until I had an acute reaction to formaldehyde from a cheap outfit purchased on-line, that I started giving all of my clothing more attention. Below is a non-exhaustive list of toxic chemicals that may be found in clothing.

Chemicals Found in Clothing:[206]

1. Doxins
2. Benzene
3. Acetic Acid

4. Dimethylformamide
5. Azo-Dyes
6. Sulfuric Acid
7. Potassium Dichromate
8. Chromium Trioxide
9. Ammonium Dichromate
10. Nonylphenol
11. Formaldehyde
12. Carbon Disulfide
13. Perfluroinated Chemicals

So why are these chemicals in our clothing in the first place and why are they bad for us? Dimethylformamide, for example, is needed to produce acrylic fibers and artificial leathers.[207] According to the CDC, when interacting directly with the skin, this chemical can cause liver damage and other adverse health effects.[208] Other chemicals such as formaldehyde are used to prevent wrinkling and shrinkage in clothing. In fact, any clothing that purports to be wrinkle, stain, or flame resistant or retardant is often treated with formaldehyde, perfluorinated chemicals (PFCs) such as Teflon, nonylphenol ethoxylates (NPEs), and nonylphenols (NPs), or triclosan.[209] NPEs and NPs are absorbable via the skin and are associated with reproductive and developmental defects in rodents. And studies have shown that factory workers regularly exposed to triclosan may have an increased cancer risk.[210] Synthetic azo dyes, commonly used for coloring clothing, leather and textiles, release amines that increased the risk of bladder cancer in German dye factory workers regularly exposed to the dyes.[211]

Speaking from my own personal experience, I purchased an outfit made in China over the internet that had clearly been treated to prevent wrinkling. I wore it directly out of the bag without washing it. Within three hours, I broke out in very severe hives that felt like burns. My skin boiled up in spots as if I'd poured acid on myself. The doctor later explained that it was very important to wash clothing before wearing it, and trust me, the lesson will not be forgotten. While the US does not regulate formaldehyde levels in clothing, the US Government Accountability Office noted that US products met the highest standards set by other countries who do regulate it.[212] The moral of my story is to always purchase clothing from reputable merchants and to always wash your clothing before wearing. A simple wash can drastically reduce the presence of these chemicals in your clothing so you are protected before wearing.

Of course, the best advice is to purchase clothing that is less likely to have chemicals on it in the first place. Cotton, silk, organic wool, hemp, alpaca, angora, camel, cashmere, mohair, flax, ramie, and aluyot are all good choices, as they are typically very minimally treated, if at all.[213]

Chemicals in Cleaning Products

At this point, it should come as no surprise that many commonly used household products contain toxic chemicals. Almost every product that purports to clean or freshen your home contains harsh chemicals and synthetic fragrances that can cause all sorts of health related issues, from asthma to cancer, skin irritations, chemical burns, and more.[214]

The Environmental Working Group tested 21 commonly used household cleaning products, from air fresheners to multi-purpose cleaning sprays, and found that they emitted over 450 chemicals into the air.[215] These chemicals included compounds linked to asthma, developmental and reproductive problems, and cancer.[216] Preservatives that release formaldehyde are commonly used in multi-purpose products.[217] Carcinogens such as 1,4-dioxane and ethylene oxide, and volatile organic compounds (VOCs) called terpenes that can react with ozone indoors to create formaldehyde may also be present in your all-purpose cleaning products.[218] Studies have shown that when pregnant mothers are exposed to such chemicals in cleaning agents, their babies may have lower birth weights, lower IQs, and respiratory symptoms throughout childhood.[219] Further, other chemicals in these products have been linked to cancer, specifically all-purpose products and dish and laundry detergents.

Worse, only about 1 in 7 products reviewed by the Environmental Working Group in 2016 fully disclosed the chemical ingredients in their products, as government regulations do not require full disclosure.[220] Often companies use generic terms such as "fragrance," or "surfactant," or "colorant," to mask dozens of hazardous chemical compound ingredients. Below are some tips from the Environmental Working Group to protect yourself from the health hazards posed by many household cleaning products.

Environmental Working Group Tips To Protect Against Harmful Cleaning Products:[221]

1. Don't use products made with triclosan, an anti-bacterial;
2. Don't use cleaners that include ammonia or chlorine bleach;
3. Don't use toilet cleaners, oven cleaners, or de-greasers that contain hydrochloric acid, phosphoric acid, sodium or potassium hydroxide, or ethanolamines;
4. Don't use air-fresheners and avoid scented cleaning and laundry products that do not disclose their fragrance ingredients;
5. Don't use products that contain quaternary ammonium compounds;
6. Look for products certified by Green Seal or Ecologo;
7. Be sure to ventilate when cleaning.

Keep it simple when cleaning your home. Whenever possible, use products such as white vinegar or water and baking soda, or even basic hot water and soap, to clean in and around your kitchens and baths when necessary. These products are effective and lack the risk of harmful side effects.

Air Quality & Radiation

Is the air around you making you sick?

Many of us spend a lot of time in air-conditioned environments, and this alone can pose health risks. Unlike heating units, air conditioning poses unique problems because the process of cooling warm air creates moisture. This moisture presents an environment for microbes to grow.[222] If your office or home air conditioning unit is not properly maintained, you could be circulating these microbes around your home or office and breathing them. Mold exposure is also a culprit in many chronic health problems, so you should ensure your home is free of it.

Electromagnetic Field radiation (EMF) can also pose a health concern. EMF radiation is not new to humans, as the sun and earth provide a natural source of EMF radiation. However, man-made EMF radiation from cell phones, cell towers, WiFi routers, microwave ovens, smart meters, etc., can cause health problems if the exposure is prolonged.[223] The International Agency for Research on Cancer has categorized low frequency EMF radiation as a class 2B possible carcinogen.[224] A recent study from the National Toxicology Program showed that high exposure to EMF radiation in rats was associated with heart tumors and evidence of brain and adrenal gland tumors.[225] Symptoms related to EMF exposure have been noted to include insomnia, anxiety, hormone imbalance, increased cancer risk, brain fog, and vertigo.[226]

It's impossible in this day in age to entirely avoid exposure to man-made EMF radiation, but you can minimize it. Shut your WiFi and cell phone off at night while you sleep. When using your cell phone, do not hold it close to your face. Instead, use speaker-phone and hold the cell phone a foot away while talking. Do not store your phone on your body when not in use. During the day if you do not need to make calls or use the internet, set your phone to airplane mode or shut it off.

Food Preparation & Storage

What you eat is just as important as *how you prepare* what you eat. Non-stick pans, plastic storage containers, plastic and aluminum wraps can be sources of unwanted chemical and heavy metal exposure.

Unfortunately, the convenience of an easy to clean non-stick frying pan can come with a few downsides. These types of pans often use poly and perfluoroalkyl substances (PFAS).[227] PFAS releases perfluorooctanoic acid (PFOA), which is a carcinogenic chemical when it is heated.[228] Non-stick pans are also often times a source of toxic heavy metals that can flake off onto your food. Aluminum and Teflon pans should also be avoided. As mentioned earlier, aluminum has been linked to Alzheimer's disease, ALS, and autism.[229] Teflon pans have a polytetrafluoroethylene coating (PTFE) that turns into toxic PFOA at high heat. Safe choices of cookware include pans from GreenLife, Scanpan, Cuisinart Green Gourmet, and GreenPan. There are others, but you must do your research.

Similarly, be leery of too much reliance upon plastic storage containers, plastic sandwich bags, aluminum foils and plastic wraps. These products can contain harmful substances, such as heavy metals, that can leach into your food.

Conclusion

I have certainly not provided an exhaustive list of ways to reduce your toxic exposure. But, surely you get the idea. We expose ourselves in unnecessary ways on a daily basis to all sorts of toxic and chemical burdens, and these substances often find their way into our bodies. I'm sure if you look around your house today you will find many sources of toxic burdens, from your WiFi to cleaning products and shampoo. Simply use common sense, check labels, and ensure the products you are using on a daily basis near and around your body are safe and simple. It is impossible to remove all sources of toxic exposure, so simply do your best. Every little thing you do on a daily basis matters and adds up over time.

CHAPTER THIRTEEN

RECOVERY STEP #8— Implement Effective Coping & Stress Management Strategies

"When we long for life without difficulties, remind us that oaks grow strong in contrary winds and diamonds are made under pressure."
Peter Marshall

A chronic and debilitating illness can feel like being buried alive. You do not technically have a terminal disease, but you feel like you are in the midst of dying every single day. The losses are many. Obviously, the pain of feeling sick every day is enormous, but so too is the sense of total loss when you can no longer be the parent you once were, maintain a career, socialize with friends and family, or simply grocery shop. Yes, you are living, but you may feel dead inside. Keeping your head above water during the healing process is certainly challenging, but you must stay positive. How do you do this?

First, you must recognize that losing your health and all that comes with it is a traumatic event. That means, in order to start making any progress on your physical health, you must also work on your mental and emotional health. The seven stages of grief perfectly delineated the emotional journey of my illness. If you are like me, you will be able to identify with each of these stages—shock & denial, pain & guilt, anger & bargaining, depression & loneliness, upward turn, reconstruction, and acceptance. Understanding each stage and effectively working through each one will help speed along your healing process.

Second, you must learn how to be happy even when your day is, by all accounts, difficult. This isn't easy, I know. Practicing meditation, mindfulness, and focusing on gratitude will be the keys to transition you out of the pit of darkness and into a place of healing.

Let's first examine the seven stages of grief.

Seven Stages of Grief

1. Shock & Denial

Do you find yourself saying, "I cannot believe this is happening to me," on a regular basis? I would tell my mother almost daily that I felt the need to pinch myself to make sure the nightmare was real. It takes time to come to terms with your limitations, your losses, and your "new normal." Not surprisingly, shock and denial is the first step in coming to terms with your disease and all it entails.

I was stuck in this stage for many months. Developing a debilitating disease at 36 years old was something that, in my opinion, happened to *other people*. It wasn't supposed to happen *to me*. Not in a million years would I have anticipated falling sick with an illness for which doctors had no solutions. Being sent home time and again from the doctor's office with zero recourse, and faced with the certainty that my life had been permanently altered, was beyond jolting.

Overcoming your initial shock is just a waiting game. Feel the feelings, examine them, cry, talk to someone who cares for you—whatever you feel you need to do. Do not be ashamed or embarrassed. These feelings will pass in their own time as you allow them to surface, and then you will be one step closer to picking up the pieces instead of continually falling apart. I can't count how many tears I've shed throughout this ordeal, but my family can attest—it has been a lot. In fact, there are days I still get emotional over it. I've been sad, scared, angry, and despondent, you name it—I've felt it, and sometimes all at once. But remember, there is absolutely no shame in showing your emotions and working through them. In fact, to the contrary, it is critical that you allow yourself to feel and purge your emotions at your own pace.

2. Pain & Guilt

Pain and guilt are the next step in your journey to acceptance and healing. As you find yourself in bed day after day, you will begin to reflect heavily on how you got there. Thoughts of, 'I guess I deserve this,' may sink in. You will then look back on anything and everything that could have contributed in any way to your falling sick, and you may have tremendous guilt. I recall thinking, 'if only I'd not worked so many hours,' or, 'if only I'd eaten better,' or, 'if only I'd not always been so stressed out.' It never ended. I felt to blame for my body falling apart on me, like I had completely failed myself. I desperately wanted to go back in time and re-do anything that might have contributed to this result.

I also vividly remember feeling completely terrified and overwhelmed. I could not make sense of my situation, and had no idea how to fix it. I felt totally out of control. The anxiety was immense. Truly, it was the feeling of being in a plane that was spiraling into the ground. Trying to wrap my head around what was happening and why and how to fix it was too much to deal with all at once. It felt like the weight of the world on my shoulders.

If you are a parent, you may also feel tremendous feelings of pain and guilt over not being able to take care of your children as you once did.

This was a very tough topic for me, as my children were only six months and 2 years old, respectively, when I first fell sick. I missed play dates, birthday parties, trick or treating, trips to the zoo and playground, and family vacations. I did literally nothing with my children during the first few years of my illness, except the bare minimum stuff, like tucking them in at night and hugging them when they got home from school. All the rest was up to my parents and my husband to manage. I was totally bedridden and too tired to do anything else. It was not my fault, and I knew that. But, the guilt of not being able to do what almost every other parent took for granted was absolutely devastating.

You may also feel, as I did, tremendous guilt over the struggle you place on your entire family simply because you're now out of the picture. I saw how hard everyone around me was working to hold it all together, and this alone was enough to make me want to crumble. I truly hated the impact my health crisis was having on those I loved. The strain of my sudden absence from the family structure meant that everyone else around me had to pull double duty. My elderly parents had to handle all of the day-to-day care of both kids. I also needed daily special attention from those around me to just prepare a meal or get to doctor appointments. My husband worked four states away when I was at my sickest, and he had to drive five hours each way on weekends to be with us. The very last thing I ever wanted to do to my family was burden them. There was nothing I could do about it, though, except work hard to get well. That meant, allowing those around me to help even though it pained me to need them so much. I had to let go and accept where I was. Getting beyond the pain and guilt took a long time.

If you find yourself in this rut of despair and guilt, know that it is part of the healing process. Sources of emotional pain are endless when you become chronically sick, so you are only human to fall apart emotionally. And it is completely normal to feel overwhelmed. *Remember that it is okay to not have all the answers right now. They will all come to you in proper time. Getting well is a slow process.* Do not panic about what protocol you should be on or whether you are doing it all "right." Simply do what you can. You do not have to get it all right at once.

3. Anger & Bargaining

For me, the anger and bargaining stage went on for months—and to some degree, years. After the initial shock of my predicament wore off, and I truly realized the nightmare was legitimate, it made me quite angry. I would tell myself I didn't deserve this. I hadn't done anything remotely terrible enough to justify the universe's current punishment. Sickness was just not supposed to happen *to me*! I would become very angry at the sight of anyone who smoked cigarettes, for instance, or ate terribly unhealthy food and yet still functioned at a normal level.

Doctors were also a source of my wrath. For a long time, I was so hostile toward doctors that I could barely stand the sight of them at my appointments. I felt so betrayed by their indifference, lack of consideration, apathy, and total failure to find anything wrong with me for months and months on end that I took it personally. In my defense, some doctors made it very difficult not to. There were doctors who treated me very poorly for simply relaying my symptoms. It was as if they were insulted by the fact they could not do anything for me, and would therefore treat me like I was faking illness. I had one doctor in particular suggest that my pain was "psychosomatic." This comment almost sent me over the edge. If I hadn't been so exhausted and sick, I may have tackled the man. I was a person who went through law school, earned honor grades, ran four miles in 90 degree heat with my children in a jogger to get groceries *just for the fun of it*, and even ran a marathon. I was not lazy, nor did I enjoy for one minute being disabled. And the slightest hint from anyone suggesting that I was not, in fact, suffering with a *real* illness, well, that was unacceptable to me. And it made my blood boil.

Sadly, it is simply difficult to find doctors who understand these chronic illnesses very well. And even when they *do* seem to understand the problem, treatment options are not that effective. You will likely be greeted with push-back from doctors when you repeatedly complain of symptoms for which they cannot find a cause or cure. It's okay to get angry. You should get angry. But, just as with all of these emotions, you must feel the anger and then let it go. Accept that there are bad doctors out there, just as there are bad teachers, lawyers, police officers, etc. But, there *will* also be many good—and some exceptional—doctors on your journey, and you're better off focusing on gratitude toward those who help you than anger toward those who fail you miserably.

There will also be friends and family members who will doubt your illness or make light of it. This was probably the most surprising aspect of developing Lyme disease—being doubted and talked about by some people as if I was a mental case who enjoyed attention. Maybe understandably, the sheer fact that my illness took a very long time to diagnose created an opening for some to conclude I was not "really" sick. I would hear "through the grapevine" the chatter of others who, allegedly, had my best interests at heart, suggesting that I didn't "look sick," or surmising that I was "just depressed," or rolling their eyes at my "neediness." I heard, "what's wrong with her *now*?" being asked by someone who should have known better.

There will also be those who do not appreciate how much you suffer, even when they *are* well intentioned and care about you. I had one friend in particular who would talk to me like I was going through a typical every day problem, like a cold, and not, in fact, a life altering disease. Because I did not look sick in the traditional sense—my hair was not falling out, I was not in a wheel chair, I did not have a cast on my limbs, etc., it was just hard for some people to fully contemplate the scope of my problems. There were days I was able to get dressed and drag myself to social functions out of obligation. And this would lead some to assume my health was fine or that I was exaggerating my situation. But the fact was, I was in terrible shape. I would go home from the few social events I attended as fast as I could, throw on my pajamas, and go directly to bed. I never enjoyed myself, I merely gutted through in a foggy haze. I'd typically be totally relegated to bed for days or weeks following any sort of formal outing. I suffered extreme post exertion malaise, such that anything beyond eating, drinking and wandering my house in my pajamas was too much for me. Having to get properly dressed, do my hair, look presentable, and then talk to people and focus on a dialogue was absolutely overwhelming.

Others just do not and cannot fully contemplate the struggle that comes with a chronic illness such as Lyme disease, CFS, or MS, nor can they relate, to much degree, to your experience. How could they? Absent going through it, there is no reference point. It's certainly nothing you can convey in words. But regardless, I would sometimes make the mistake of vocalizing how very weak and tired I felt to whomever I was with, and the other person would often respond with, "yeah I'm tired too." And yes, the comparison of my bone-crushing exhaustion to the everyday tiredness of being a working parent upset me. They were just two different things. Some days, being so misunderstood upset me a lot more than it should have. I did not enjoy feeling like I had to explain myself or *prove* to others that I was sick. But, I did. And that's just the way it was, and it may very well be the case for you. And that's ok!

You've simply got to remember during your journey to get well, the opinions, casual assessments, and comments of others are inconsequential. They mean nothing and are not your concern. Let others say and think what they want; they don't understand your situation. For the most part, people mean well, they just cannot understand what they have never personally experienced. As for those who go out of their way to treat you poorly, well, that is a reflection on them and not you. Frankly, their ignorant and hurtful comments expose them for who they really are, and that in itself is a gift. The people who hurt you likely have their own sets of problems to work through. Their behavior is a symptom of a deeper problem within themselves. Forgive them. They are on a journey too.

Your focus while healing should always be on gratitude and the love you feel toward those who are helping you. Look around you right now, and identify all you have to be grateful for. I bet there is a lot. You've likely got a roof over your head, a bed to sleep in, food to eat, and people in your life who love you. Anger will not serve you well for very long, so you must let it go. It's like an anchor around your feet holding you back. To get well, you've got to let go of all the things that weigh you down, and anger is heavy.

Remember, you may be sick, but you are alive. And now you are on the path to getting well. *That* is something to be happy about!

4. Depression, Reflection, and Loneliness
This stage of grief needs little explanation. Having a debilitating illness that takes virtually everything away from you is obviously going to cause a depressed mood and feelings of loneliness. Losing your career, your ability to socialize and partake in life like a normal person is decimating on your emotional state. Medical doctors would often ask me if I was depressed in my appointments, and I thought it was such an odd question. Of course I was depressed. Who wouldn't be? I was living with my mother and father with an illness that no one could cure. Is there a person who would not be depressed? The difference, though, was that if my circumstances could have changed overnight, I'd have been the happiest person on the planet and ready to jump back into life. I was not clinically depressed. But I was certainly lonely and despondent.

Going through a prolonged illness is so very isolating, as few people can relate to your situation. Simply carrying on a conversation with someone and being understood is next to impossible. It feels like absolutely no one "gets" it. And because you are sick for so long, most people get tired of hearing you complain day-in and day-out about your problems. So, you start to keep it to yourself. Pretty soon you are living in your own head 24 hours a day. It's a lonely place.

I wish there was a magic wand to make these feelings of depression and isolation go away, but they simply need to be felt. I truly believe it is necessary to feel these difficult emotions so that you can bottom out. By all means, though, if you are feeling suicidal or truly clinically depressed, be sure to seek a doctor's consult right away. But, the sadness and general depression that come with feeling defeated by your situation is something you will have to sit with until it becomes so intolerable that you let it go. You can only stay depressed for so long, before you realize it's time to stop sulking. You'll get to the point where enough is enough and being a victim no longer suits you. When you get to this point, everything will shift, and you will begin the long and slow process of turning it around.

5. Upward Turn

Every great story has its turning point. Yours will have one too. In Rocky II, it's the moment where Adrian tells Rocky to win. Suddenly, Rocky snaps out of his mental fog and depression and becomes inspired to fight again. Your turning point will come after you've bottomed out and purged yourself of so many emotions that you can barely feel anything anymore.

The period just before my upward turn was a bit like being on a road trip where I was so wiped out, nothing bothered me. I was simply numb to the pain. Sick and tired of being sick and tired, with nowhere to go, I found myself at a crossroads. I was reminded of the scene in Shawshank Redemption where the character Red says, "life comes down to a simple choice: You're either busy living or busy dying." Precisely. The choice is always yours.

Are you going to get to work healing or are you going to wallow in anger, self-defeat and pity and give up? Being a mother to two small children who needed me, I wasn't going to quit. I made a pledge to myself that from there on out, I was going to do everything and anything to get myself well. Whatever it took, I would do it.

At this point, I was certainly still deep in despair, but my focus became the solution rather than the devastation. I began to research heavily both on-line and in any book on chronic illness that I could get my hands on. I'd watch webinars and TEDx talks and anything that discussed healing the body from a chronic illness. Eventually, I also aligned myself with practitioners who were better suited to help a person with chronic disease.

Don't get me wrong, it is not all roses and smooth sailing once you hit your turning point. In fact, it is the total opposite. There will be countless low points along the way before you get well. You will have continual, periodic and cyclic setbacks that will feel devastating. Some of those setbacks may last a long time. But your overall trajectory from this point onward will be up—even if minimally and you struggle to see it.

6. Reconstruction & Working Through
In a word, this period of your healing is all about empowerment. When you're truly sick of being sick, you will get very serious about everything you do relative to your body and health. Committed to getting well, you will start to implement your protocol with faith and determination. And you will begin to believe that you *can* get yourself better, that you have the power *within you* to heal, and that you need only to properly support your body.

Maybe you have found an excellent doctor or practitioner at this point or you are simply implementing *The Wahls Protocol* with laser precision. But this period is all about finding what works for you and implementing it with fierce devotion. You will begin the inner work needed to recover without the frenetic worry you felt in the earlier stages of your illness. You will be running with blinders on, not burdening yourself with doubt and worry, but instead focusing on your protocol and putting one foot in front of the other.

This is a difficult stage of the healing process, because you will likely have repeated healing crises. If you suffer from Lyme disease, you probably already know what I am talking about. Often as you are getting better, you go through periods where you feel much worse. This is typically because you are experiencing a "die off" reaction due to the herbal protocols you are taking or simply from changing your diet from one of processed foods and sugar to one of primarily vegetables and low to no sugar. Your body is going to be transitioning back into balance, and you will feel all sorts of symptoms along the way. If you are like me, you will go periods where you are quite sure you are improving, only to get slammed backward out of the blue for a week or two (or three or four!). But you will start to notice that every time you come out of a downturn, you will be slightly better than you were before.

Always stay calm and assured when you hit these inevitable setbacks. Every person who gets well goes through this same thing. You will have moments of extreme doubt. But do not lose hope. Stick to your protocols and good habits. Be unrelenting in your desire to get well and do the heavy lifting of eating properly, even when all seems lost. You will come out of the proverbial death spiral. It's simply a matter of time and taking care of your body, allowing it to rest and regroup. If your healing crisis is particularly difficult, go off all of your supplements for a period. I did this quite frequently. Hopefully, you are able to work with an experienced practitioner who can walk you through these difficult times, but if you are not, simply listen to your body. You know when your body needs a break. Don't push too hard.

Imagine running a marathon. The reconstruction period is the point in which you come into your stride, you've got a good chunk of mileage behind you, but still a long road ahead. But you're on your way! Stay the course, no matter what, and pat yourself on the back for all of your efforts. Getting well is hard work!

7. Acceptance

One of my favorite quotes, and one that is truly reflective of this stage in the healing process, is by A.A. Milne, the author of the famous Winnie the Pooh books. It reads:

"What day is it?' asked Pooh.
"It's today," squeaked Piglet.
"My favorite day," said Pooh.

Acceptance means you finally realize you are okay right where you are, no matter your circumstances. Even when you feel terrible, it is possible to be happy, content, and grateful. Illness may feel like a curse, but life itself—with all of its difficulties and ups and downs—is an incredible gift. We are not promised tomorrow. Living for today, no matter how terrible you may feel, is what we all must do. And be honest; no one has a perfect life. Even the people who appear to have it all—good health, happiness, a fulfilling career and family—those people have problems too. The secret to happiness and contentment is *not* in getting well. It is in *choosing* to be grateful and loving toward yourself and others in all ways and at all times. And ironically, choosing to feel this way, despite being so sick, will help you to heal faster!

Another lesson I've learned is that not many things ever work out exactly as planned, and that is okay. As I discussed earlier, a difficult sticking point for me was my failure to be the mom I'd always envisioned. When I first had kids, I envisioned playing soccer in the yard, taking them on vacations to the beach, going on long bike rides to the park, and being very actively involved with them. So, when I fell sick and had to miss out on virtually all of their toddler and pre-school years (and a lot of the elementary years as well), it was all the more devastating to me. I kept comparing myself to the fictional mother I'd created in my mind, and I simply did not measure up. Don't do that to yourself.

Accept your life for what it is and where you are. While I was busy berating myself for not being a perfect mother, my kids were enjoying their lives. They had grandparents who doted on them, two loving parents who were always there for them, aunts, uncles, and cousins who were actively a part of their lives. And although I was sick, my kids would watch movies with me in bed, see me every day when they got home from school, and never felt anything was amiss. They felt loved and safe. And that was all that mattered. In fact, I actually *was* being a good mom. Even when I was at my worst, I still ensured all of their needs were met. If I had been honest with myself, I'd have acknowledged that I was being a *great* mom. There had been no reason to beat myself up at all. But, I did simply because of a faux expectation I'd created in my head.

There are reasons you may not yet understand as to why you need to experience this difficulty. There are lessons you need to learn and tools you need to gain from this experience. What those lessons are exactly is up to you to discover. Everyone is different. Embrace all of the lessons, as they are the silver lining to your storm clouds. These hardships are going to make you a better person in the end. You are going to come out of illness with a strength you never knew you had and a unique perspective on what it means to be well—things most people fail to achieve in their lifetime. And when you reach this point, think about what you will do with your "new" self. Perhaps you will go out into the world and help someone else who needs it, just as you needed it in the pits of illness.

When you progress to the acceptance stage, you may also find that you are not constantly cursing the world for your illness. This is a good thing, because as the saying goes, what you resist persists. Letting go of your resistance to illness is exactly what your body needs to get well. Learn to be okay with being sick. That doesn't mean settle in and set up shop. It means recognize being sick as a mere stop along the way to the place you are ultimately going. I am not a particularly religious person, but I do believe in God. And I always felt in my heart that if I simply did all that I could on my end to improve my situation, that God and the universe would meet me half-way. And I let it go at that. If I knew I was doing all I could do in the moment and throughout the day, then I gave the rest of my worries to God to handle.

All you can do at any given time is your best. *So simply do your best.* Stick to your protocol, love yourself enough to be strict with your diet, and hold tightly to your faith. Then let go, relax, and enjoy your life.

Meditation, Mindfulness, & Gratitude

Maintaining this healthy perspective will take work, because you will have setbacks in your health, life problems will arise, and there will simply always be obstacles popping up to test your resolve. It's important to actively train your brain to stay mindful and calm in the face of adversity. Don't chase the rabbit down the hole every time a potential problem arises, or a "what-if" question presents itself. I have been guilty of "what iffing" myself almost to death. Any time a symptom would reemerge, I'd immediately think—what if it's back? What if this time I fall backward and can't get out of it? It's normal to have these thoughts. But don't dwell on them. They are lies. Your body is in the process of healing, and your body will do the work. Your job is to get out of its way, stay in the present moment, remain calm, and let your body do its job. Don't use up valuable energy worrying. Being mindful will help you do this.

The absolute best way to practice mindfulness is to begin a daily meditation practice. There are some excellent meditation applications you can download, one in particular is called 10% Happier. Meditation will help you calm your thoughts, and over time it conditions your brain to not overreact. If sitting and meditating is not your thing, use your daily walks as a source of calm and quiet reflection. Make a point each day to be alone and quiet your mind, and simply notice all that is around you. I would sit and do meditation exercises each morning before I was able to go for walks. Now, I view my daily walks or runs as meditation. I don't go with anyone else. It is my peaceful, quiet time for myself.

I also recommend reading uplifting books such as daily devotionals. My favorite daily devotional is called, "Jesus Calling," by Sarah Young. Each day, this book presents a scripture with the author's interpretation and relevance to our everyday lives. Sarah Young has also battled Lyme disease, and I know her writing is inspired by her experiences. Everyone who goes through a chronic illness at some point needs a cheerleader. This book serves that purpose. I have used it daily for several years now.

Maintaining a proper mindset is sometimes less about what you should do, and more about what you should not do. One of the most important things you should *not* do while getting well is join every single Facebook group out there on chronic illness. These groups can be fantastic resources, but you must choose them wisely. I found that the vast majority of Lyme disease and chronic illness groups amounted to a mass of sick people constantly venting about how horrible their lives had become. I am not blaming any of these people for needing an outlet. They were (and are) all legitimately suffering. But constantly reading about other peoples' problems and every single protocol they are trying will drain you emotionally and physically. Certainly, if you have a question about something you are going through, log on and ask. But do not make a habit of reading through the daily postings of these sites. They will only bring you down. You must take care of yourself right now. Sadly, there are some people who truly enjoy complaining about their illness all of the time, even when it's unnecessary. Don't step unwittingly into their quicksand. Chronic Lyme disease, in particular, is very tough to recover from. To beat it, you have to stay positive and focused. What I needed while sick was a pick-me-up, not a weight on my ankles. So, I left all but a very few select groups. Gravitate toward the forums where people share their success stories. Those stories will be the wind in your sails.

Conclusion

You must be positive and determined in order to get well. Coping "well" is a learned skill and does not just happen. You must be proactive in your fight to keep the thoughts in your head productive and positive. That does not mean refusing to have a negative thought or never having a bad day. It means staying committed to working toward your goal. If you fall off the horse, get back on it. If you have a day of anger, despair, and frustration, start over again tomorrow. Just do not give up. For the most part, the difference between the people who get well and those who do not is mindset. Work through your emotions, but do not drown in them.

CHAPTER FOURTEEN

FINDING A PRACTITONER & RELIABLE RESOURCES

"The strong individual is the one who asks for help when he needs it."
Rona Barrett

We are so very lucky to live in this modern era with access to the internet and endless amounts of information. I often thought about what I would have done had I gotten sick prior to the internet and Facebook. Being able to research so easily at home in bed made the process of getting well so much easier. Hopefully, my years of researching can streamline the process for you. As the saying goes, you have to kiss a lot of frogs to find your prince. I met with a seemingly endless number of doctors and practitioners who were, frankly, worthless before I found resources that actually yielded results. In this chapter, I list for you the practitioners and resources I consider to be the best of the best.

Skype Practitioners

If you are unable to find functional medicine practitioners in your area, there are many practitioners who offer Skype consultations. Skype consultations are an enormous help when you are too sick to leave your house. I also found Skype consultations to be much more beneficial than face-to-face office visits, as more time was spent discussing my situation.

I wish my list of Skype practitioners was lengthier, but the five below are top-notch. This does not mean there are not others who are equally qualified. Research on-line and check out their reviews. There are many LLMDs throughout the country as well, but I have not listed any below. This is simply because I did not find them terribly useful in my recovery. However, every case is different, and you may, in fact, need a LLMD. Facebook Lyme disease forums can be a huge help in finding a reputable LLMD, as you can get insightful feedback and reviews directly from other Lyme patients.

1. **Jennifer Sierzant, Certified Naturopath** – Jennifer has been my naturopath for many years now. She is very caring and has a deep appreciation for chronic illness, as she suffered through Lyme disease and lupus for many years. She is located in Quebec, Canada, but does Skype consultations internationally. She can help you with virtually any ailment, but she is especially versed in Lyme and autoimmune disease treatments. Her web address is: https://www.jennifersierzant.com.

2. **Dr. Justin Marchegiani, D.C. / Just In Health Wellness Clinic** – Dr. Justin was an excellent resource for me. He performed state-of-the-art testing that was on-par or better than what was offered at the Cleveland Clinic Functional Medicine program. Only, Dr. Justin was available from the comfort of my own home via Skype at a fraction of the cost. He has a heavy presence on Facebook and offers many webinars with question and answer sessions that are very informative. His web address is: https://justinhealth.com.

3. **Katina Makris, C.C.H., C.I.H.** – Katina Makris is a Certified Homeopath, Certified Intuitive Healer, and author who specializes in Lyme disease. She personally suffered with Lyme disease for many years, and I found her to be a tremendous resource. She offers phone consultations and is also the author of several books on overcoming Lyme and chronic illness. Her web address is: https://katinamakris.com.

4. **Dr. Gary Gruber, Naturopathic Physician** – Dr. Gary Gruber is a naturopathic doctor who practices in New Canaan and Stamford, Connecticut. He treats patients with acute and chronic illnesses, such as Lyme, CFS, and autoimmune disease among others. He is available for remote conferencing (he does not use Skype, but another form of video conferencing that is HIPAA compliant), and he has many positive patient reviews. His web address is: www.sciencemeetsnature.org.

5. **Lone Pedersen, D.C.H., M.N.H.L.** – Lone Pedersen practices homeopathy, and she specializes in anxiety, depression, OCD and ADHD, although she does also work with patients who suffer CFS. I currently work with her to help heal my thyroid and improve my energy. I also work with her for my son who, like many children, can have problems concentrating at school. Lone has been tremendously helpful to our family, and I recommend her highly. She has many clients who have reported total reversals in chronic anxiety and depression, both of which can be major problems for those suffering a chronic illness. Her web address is: https://www.naturligvishomeopathy.com.

Must-Read Books

Do not ever stop learning from other people's experiences. Read the personal accounts of others who have recovered from chronic illness, and the accounts of those who have successfully treated patients with chronic illness. Each account will be slightly different, and you will pick up a wealth of useful tips and advice. We are all very unique individuals with unique biology, so what worked for one person may not work for another. Keep an open mind and learn from others who have walked the path before you.

My Favorite Must-Read Books:

1. *The Wahls Protocol: How I Beat Progressive MS Using Paleo Principles and Functional Medicine*, by Terry Wahls, M.D.;

2. *The Lyme Solution: A Five-Part Plan to Fight the Inflammatory Autoimmune Response and Beat Lyme Disease*, by Darin Ingels, N.D., F.A.A.E.M.;

3. *Gut Health Protocol: A Nutritional Approach to Healing SIBO, Intestinal Candida, GERD, Gastritis, and other Gut Health Issues*, by John G. Herron;

4. *Unlocking Lyme: Myths, Truths, and Practical Solutions for Chronic Lyme Disease*, by William Rahls, M.D.;

5. *Out of the Woods: Healing from Lyme Disease for Body, Mind and Spirit*, by Katina Makris, C.C.H., C.I.H.;

6. *Why Can't I Get Better? Solving the Mystery of Lyme & Chronic Disease*, by Dr. Richard Horowitz;

7. *Stop the Thyroid Madness: A Patient Revolution Against Decades of Inferior Treatment*, by Janie A. Bowthorpe;

8. *Why Do I Still Have Thyroid Symptoms? When My Lab Tests Are Normal: A Revolutionary Breakthrough in Understanding Hashimoto's Disease and Hypothyroidism*, by Dr. Datis Kharrazian.

My Favorite On-line Resources

1. **Treat Lyme by Marty Ross MD (www.treatlyme.net)** – Dr. Marty Ross treated me via Skype early in my illness. I found him to be quite knowledgeable in Lyme disease and chronic fatigue syndrome. His practice has changed, however, and he now offers a web-site with direct and free access to treatment protocols, including videos. This is obviously a great resource for anyone with financial restraints who cannot afford a practitioner.

2. **MS Saved My Life (www.mssavedmylife.com)** – Natalie reversed MS using diet, and she discusses how she eats to maintain her health. Natalie also developed a line of non-toxic and natural skin care products. I have enjoyed following her throughout the years and have gained a lot of great tips, especially when it comes to diet, from her posts.

3. **Real Food Rebel (www.realfoodrebel.com)** – Brenda Cosentino recovered from chronic Lyme disease, CFS, and fibromyalgia among other things. Her site is a treasure trove of great information. She is also a Nutritional Therapy Consultant.

4. **Real Food Inspired Me (www.bethschultz.com)** – Beth Schultz reversed MS and Lyme disease using diet, and she currently works as a Nutritional Therapy Practitioner. She has a heavy presence on Facebook as well. She is incredibly inspiring and has found a lot of success following *The Wahls Protocol*. She is an excellent resource for anyone struggling with Lyme or autoimmune disease.

5. **Multiple Sclerosis Journey with Carolyn n Ron (www.justaripple.org and on Facebook at www.facebook.com/CarolynnRons)** – Dr. Ronald Girard chronicles his success fighting MS with *The Wahls Protocol*. He has an excellent Facebook page where he frequently posts candid videos sharing his incredibly inspirational journey in real-time. Dr. Girard is a tremendous source of information.

Conclusion

These resources have been enormously helpful for me, but obviously there are infinite sources of new information each and every day. Be curious and open-minded on your path to getting well. But also be dubious, as there are many companies and doctors out there selling snake oil purported to provide a quick fix. I've found that when a supplement, product, or practitioner promises the world, you can almost guaranty failure. Chronically sick people, sadly, are a target for marketers looking to sell the latest and greatest quick fixes, which I promise almost never work. Be smart about where you spend your money and in whose hands you place your trust. There is no quick and easy path to getting well. Anyone who claims otherwise is a charlatan. I've found the resources above to be very reliable.

CHAPTER FIFTEEN

FINAL WORDS

"What lies behind us and what lies before us are tiny matters compared to what lies within us."
Ralph Waldo Emerson

People very often ask me, "are you better yet?" This question always gives me pause, as I'm never quite certain how to answer it. Yes, I am doing better. Yes, I am no longer bedridden. Yes, I am able to live a fulfilling life and attend my children's activities and enjoy social events. Yes, I feel 100% better than I did five years ago. But this notion of being "better" is a slippery thing. What does it actually mean?

What I've come to realize is that I will never be 100% better, because I am always looking for ways to improve my health. That won't change, even as I am able to do more and more things. I'm finding that focusing on true health, not fad diets, or magic pills or supplements meant to cure specific ailments, makes me feel better and better with each passing day, month, and year. I am constantly honing what I do each day, mentally, physically, and spiritually, to improve my health. So, I am always in the process of "getting better." When will I be done getting better? Never! I am almost excited to see how I feel when I hit 60 years old, because I suspect I will be feeling "better" than almost all of my contemporaries simply due to how I now eat and care for myself.

How you and I feel today in this moment is simply relative to how we felt yesterday. If we are doing it all right and taking good care of our bodies, we should always be feeling better with each passing day. Of course you will have ups and downs on this path, and some days it may not be quite clear where you are on the spectrum of health. But generally speaking, if you adhere to the principles in this book, you will start to make improvements—maybe very small ones at first that even you cannot see. But those close to you will see them. And, eventually you will too. Whether at some point you and I hit a ceiling of diminishing returns, well, that may happen. With age, we all decline to some degree. That is inevitable. But there is no reason any of us should succumb to illness or the idea that with age comes poor health. It doesn't need to be that way.

I certainly still have days where I can't do much. But I also now have days where I am out jogging again, playing soccer in the summer heat with my daughter, and speed walking my neighborhood. And while none of this has ever been about weight loss or appearance, I now weigh less in my 40's than I did as a senior in high school. Yet, I never diet; I simply eat properly, and in so doing, I remain at a proper and healthy weight year after year. My trajectory is upward, and I'm not looking back.

From this day forward, you need to view *your* trajectory as upward. No more wallowing in pity and despair. Take control of your situation and get focused. Follow the recommendations I've set forth, and expect to get well.

Also, do not let money stand in the way of progress. Some chronically sick people get very discouraged when they find out the cost of functional medicine appointments and testing, as these appointments are not typically covered by insurance. This alone makes them feel defeated and hopeless from the outset. If you can't afford a practitioner or fancy supplements, do not throw in the towel. You can go very far on diet alone—in fact, I dare say you can probably go all the way. If organic food is too expensive for your budget, simply opt for non-organic vegetables and fruits. They are far less expensive and will still get you results. Supplements, herbal protocols, antibiotics, and fancy expensive testing may be helpful, but they might be totally unnecessary. You may find that by simply following the nutritional principles I've outlined in this book, you can reverse your symptoms on your own with food.

Remember, the decisions you make from minute-to-minute about what to eat will have the largest impact on your outcome. Yes, there are people who regain their health from illnesses such as Lyme disease through antibiotics while never changing their diets. But, Lyme disease can come back. And other diseases can also pop up. If you continue with a poor diet, eating carbohydrates with reckless abandon and sugar, you will inevitably fall backward and end up sick again down the road. Your diet is the foundation for everything. Nothing else is even remotely as important or as powerful. There are no herbal protocols or supplements or medicines or expensive doctors or elite hospitals that compare to the power of proper nutrition. None. ***So, do not allow yourself any excuses for eating poorly!***

Your mindset will also be a key indicator of your success. What we focus on, we manifest. Are you going to manifest health or sickness? That will largely depend on your daily thoughts. Are you envisioning yourself getting well, tasting it, feeling it, expecting it, planning for it? Or, are you resigned to the status quo of barely getting by and expecting the worst? I do not know your specific set of circumstances, but I do know people who were far more sick than I ever was who reversed their illnesses using the principles I've set forth in this book. These incredible people refused to accept their illnesses as proverbial death sentences and committed, like true warriors, to doing whatever was in their power to get well. They pictured themselves well, even while sick and wheelchair bound. They believed, at the core of their being, that they were healing each day—whether their bodies confirmed this feeling or not.

Please read the stories of the people I listed in the former chapter and get inspired. If Dr. Ronald Girard, for example, can get up every day and fight MS as he does, you can fight whatever you are battling today too. I know it is hard. But you must stay motivated and believe in yourself. I won't lie, there were days when I felt like throwing in the towel and frankly wasn't sure I was going to live much longer. But even when I felt this way, I stuck to my core protocol and kept moving. If I was going to die, I was going to die trying to get well. You will have many days where you don't feel like a warrior or a champion, but you must always pick yourself up and keep going. Get a daily devotional and follow inspiring people on social media who are out there winning their battles against chronic illness. There are many people out there like Dr. Girard, Beth Schultz, Katina Makris, or Dr. Terry Wahls who will deeply inspire and motivate you to keep going when times are tough. Picture yourself getting well, meditate on it. Envision what your life will look like when you are feeling better. Whatever your brain focuses on, your body will gravitate toward. Be sure your focus is on health and not illness!

I would also like to point out that I experimented with *many* protocols to regain my health, and I left many of them out of this book. From RIFE machines to pulsed electromagnetic field (PEMF) mats, kinesiology, the salt C protocol, IVs of various vitamin cocktails, and antibiotic regimens … I won't say I've tried everything out there, but I've tried a lot of them. In this book, I've presented what I found to work *for me*. I'm not saying these other modalities do not work, but they did not significantly contribute to my success.

Accepting Help

To get well, I needed help, not just from practitioners but from my family. And you will need help and support as well. The complete irony is that often people suffering with invisible and chronic illnesses are viewed by others as lazy or dramatic types who exaggerate their symptoms, and therefore do not truly need help. Meanwhile, nothing could be further from the truth. I can assure you, nothing has ever demanded of me the herculean effort that chronic Lyme, CFS, and autoimmune disease has required. By the time I finally cried mercy and moved in with my parents, I'd struggled and pushed through an enormous amount of pain and fatigue on my own. I simply could not do it anymore.

If you find yourself in a similar situation, do not guilt yourself for requiring help from those around you. Accept their help with gratitude. Cast aside any judgments that may befall upon you from outsiders. They do not know your struggle or understand it, so they are certainly in no place to judge it. Then pat yourself on the back every single day you continue to battle your illness like a champion, because you deserve it. If I could give every one of you suffering through chronic illness a trophy for your efforts, I would. But the real prize will be regaining your health.

The Only Way Out is Through

Robert Frost once wrote, *"[h]e says the best way out is always through. And I can agree with that, or in so far as that I can see no way out but through."*

There is no simple way out of a chronic and debilitating illness. There are no shortcuts and no magic pills. There is only your determination, perseverance, and relentless devotion when times are terribly difficult to get you through. And times *are* going to be difficult—maybe seemingly impossible. But don't give up on yourself. Life is a beautiful thing, and this journey you are on can yield a lot of wonderful gifts, if you allow it.

Choose to be happy, regardless of your circumstances. Commit to looking at illness as a learning experience from which to grow. Do not view it as a permanent place of suffering. This is where you find yourself today, but it's not where you are headed. Tell yourself that health is coming, expect it, and know where you are now is merely a stop along the way.

Let today be the first day of the rest of your life. Keep the faith, and never stop moving forward. You deserve nothing less than a life of happiness and good health!

Consultations & Contact Information

Lastly, I offer personal consultations to anyone who would like to discuss in more detail any of the steps I took to regain my health. I am constantly learning, trying new foods and herbal protocols, and striving for excellent health. So much of what I've gone through was left out of this book due to space constraints. In a phone or Skype consultation, we can discuss more deeply any area in which you struggle.

I want to emphasize, I am not a doctor and cannot offer any sort of medical advice, evaluation, treatment, or diagnosis. However, I am happy to help you bounce ideas, offer suggestions to discuss with your doctor, and help get you going in the right direction.

For More Information Visit:

Email:
info@thehealerwithin.me

Web-Site:
www.thehealerwithin.me

Facebook:
The Healer Within/ https://www.facebook.com/thehealerwithinyou

Instagram:
The Healer Within

ENDNOTES

1. CDC Centers for Disease Control and Prevention. *Post-treatment Lyme Disease Syndrome.* Retrieved from URL: https://www.cdc.gov/lyme/postlds/index.html. See also, National Center for Biotechnology Information (NCBI) / PubMed.gov. *Chronic Lyme Disease.* Retrieved from URL: National Center for Biotechnology Information (NCBI) / PubMed.gov.
2. Holtfort Medical Group. *How Does Lyme disease Evade the Immune System?* Retrieved from URL: https://www.holtorfmed.com/lyme-disease-evade-immune-system.
3. See above.
4. See above.
5. Rawls MD. *Lyme + Herxheimer Reactions Your Guide to Feeling Good Again.* (2019, January 21). Retrieved from URL: https://rawlsmd.com/health-articles/lyme-herxheimer-reactions-your-guide-to-feeling-good-again.
6. Lyme disease Association, Inc. *Cases, Stats, Maps, & Graphs.* (2013, August 27). Retrieved from URL: https://www.lymediseaseassociation.org/about-lyme/cases-stats-maps-a-graphs/940-lyme-in-more-than-80-countries-worldwide.
7. CDC Centers for Disease Control and Prevention. *Lyme disease.* (2018, January). Retrieved from URL: https://www.cdc.gov/lyme/index.html.
8. CDC Centers for Disease Control and Prevention. *Tickborne Disease of the United States.* (2017, July 25). Retrieved from URL: https://www.cdc.gov/ticks/diseases/index.html.
9. PBS News Hour. *Self-cloning Asian tick causing worry in New Jersey.* (2018, May 26). Retrieved from URL: https://www.pbs.org/newshour/science/self-cloning-asian-tick-causing-worry-in-new-jersey.
10. Johnson, L. *Two-tiered Lab Testing for Lyme disease—No Better Than a Coin Toss. Time For Change?* (2014, October 9). Retrieved from lymedisease.

org URL: https://www.lymedisease.org/lymepolicywonk-two-tiered-lab-testing-for-lyme-disease-no-better-than-a-coin-toss-time-for-change-2.

[11] Thompson, D. *Lyme disease is vastly under-reported, CDC says.* (2015, August 12). Retrieved from URL: https://www.cbsnews.com/news/lyme-disease-more-common-cdc-says. See also, Skerret, P.. *Lyme disease 10 times more common than thought.* (2013, August 20). Retrieved from URL: https://www.health.harvard.edu/blog/lyme-disease-10-times-more-common-than-thought-201308206621.

[12] Johnson, L. *Misdiagnosis of Lyme disease as MS – MyLymeData Quick Bytes.* (2016, April 19). Retrieved from URL: https://www.lymedisease.org/lymepolicywonk-lyme-neurologic-misdiagnosis.

[13] CDC Centers for Disease Control and Prevention. *May 12 is ME/CFS and Fibromyalgia International Awareness Day.* (2018, May 10). Retrieved from URL: https://www.cdc.gov/features/cfsawarenessday/index.html; See also, CDC Centers for Disease Control and Prevention. *Fibromyalgia.* (2018, April 3). Retrieved from URL: https://www.cdc.gov/arthritis/basics/fibromyalgia.htm.

[14] CDC Centers for Disease Control and Prevention. *Myalgic Enchephalomyelitis/Chronic Fatigue Syndrome.* (2018, April 27). Retrieved from URL: https://www.cdc.gov/me-cfs/index.html; See also, CDC Centers for Disease Control and Prevention. *Fibromyalgia.* (2018, April 3). Retrieved from URL: https://www.cdc.gov/arthritis/basics/fibromyalgia.htm.

[15] American Autoimmune Related Diseases Association. *Growing Number of Autoimmune Disease Cases Reported.* (2012, June 21). Retrieved from URL: https://www.newswise.com/articles/growing-number-of-autoimmune-disease-cases-reported.

[16] WebMD. *What Are Autoimmune Disorders?* (2016, August 7). Retrieved from URL: https://www.webmd.com/a-to-z-guides/autoimmune-diseases.

[17] See above.

[18] See above.

[19] Rawls MD. *What Causes Aging & Disease.* (2016, October 20). Retrieved from URL: https://rawlsmd.com/health-articles/seven-main-causes-disease. See also, *The Wahls Protocol*, by Terry Wahls, M.D. New York: Penguin Group, 2014, pp. 46-47. See also, Marcheggiani, T., N.D. *9 Root Causes of Disease.* Retrieved from URL: https://www.bettercare.online/disease.

20. Carr, T. *Too Many Meds? America's Love Affair with Prescription Medication.* (2017, August 3). Retrieved from Consumer Reports URL: https://www.consumerreports.org/prescription-drugs/too-many-meds-americas-love-affair-with-prescription-medication.

21. Rawls MD. *What Causes Aging & Disease.* (2016, October 20). Retrieved from URL: https://rawlsmd.com/health-articles/seven-main-causes-disease.

22. See above.

23. *The Wahls Protocol*, by Terry Wahls, M.D. New York: Penguin Group, 2014, pg. 47

24. Amy Myers, M.D. *The Leaky Gut and Autoimmune Connection.* Retrieved from URL: https://www.amymyersmd.com/2017/10/leaky-gut-autoimmune-connection.

25. See above.

26. See above.

27. Health Line. *Is Leaky Gut Syndrome a Real Condition? An Unbiased Look.* (2017, February 2). Retrieved from URL: https://www.healthline.com/nutrition/is-leaky-gut-real.

28. Grisanti, R., D.C., D.A.B., C.O., D.A.C.B.N., M.S. *Leaky Gut: Can This Be Destroying Your Health?* Retrieved from URL: https://www.functionalmedicineuniversity.com/public/Leaky-Gut.cfm.

29. GI Society. *Debunking the Myth of 'Leaky Gut Syndrome.'* Retrieved from URL: https://www.badgut.org/information-centre/a-z-digestive-topics/leaky-gut-syndrome.

30. See above.

31. National Center for Biotechnology Information (NCBI) / PubMed.gov. *Gut Bacteria in Health and Disease.* (2013, September 9). Retrieved from URL: https://www.ncbi.nlm.nih.gov/pmc/articles/PMC3983973.

32. National Center for Biotechnology Information (NCBI) / PubMed.gov. *Gut Bacteria in Health and Disease.* (2013, September 9). Retrieved from URL: https://www.ncbi.nlm.nih.gov/pmc/articles/PMC3983973. See also, California Institute of Technology. *Microbes Help Produce Serotonin in Gut.* Retrieved from URL: http://www.caltech.edu/news/microbes-help-produce-serotonin-gut-46495. See also, John Hopkins Medical. *The Gut: Where Bacteria and Immune System Meet.* Retrieved from URL: https://www.hopkinsmedicine.org/research/advancements-in-research/fundamentals/in-depth/the-gut-where-bacteria-and-immune-system-meet.

33. Cell Press. *Recirculating Intestinal IgA-Producing Cells Regulate Neuroinflammation via IL-10.* (2019, January 3). Retrieved from URL: https://www.cell.com/cell/fulltext/S0092-8674(18)31560-5?fbclid=IwAR2ijfwgjurs0_CT3FwYzDi1jWtDk0bB75Eu9Ho2TPyShafdWgmlt5wGeI8.

34. California Institute of Technology. *Microbes Help Produce Serotonin in Gut.* Retrieved from URL: http://www.caltech.edu/news/microbes-help-produce-serotonin-gut-46495.

35. NYU Langone Health Division of Gastroenterology, Department of Medicine. *Your Gut Feeling: A Healthier Digestive System Means a Healthier You.* Retrieved from URL: https://med.nyu.edu/medicine/gastro/about-us/gastroenterology-news-archive/your-gut-feeling-healthier-digestive-system-means-healthier.

36. *The Wahls Protocol*, by Terry Wahls, M.D. New York: Penguin Group, 2014.

37. Hyberbiotics. *The 9 Very Worst Foods and Drinks for Your Immune System.* Retrieved from URL: https://www.hyperbiotics.com/blogs/recent-articles/the-very-worst-foods-and-drinks-for-your-immune-system.

38. Jockers, D., D.N.M., D.C., M.S. *What Is Gluten and Why Is It So Bad?* Retrieved from URL: https://drjockers.com/gluten-bad.

39. See above.

40. See above.

41. Nutriciously. *The Casein Cancer Link or Why You Should Ditch That Milk For Good.* (2016, October 24). Retrieved from URL: https://nutriciously.com/casein-cancer-connection.

42. See above.

43. See above.

44. Dr. Will Cole. *Should You Be Taking L-Glutamine for Your Gut Health?* (2018, January 11). Retrieved from URL: https://drwillcole.com/taking-l-glutamine-gut-health. See also_Dr. Axe Food is Medicine. *L-Glutamine Benefits Leaky Gut & Metabolism.* (2018, April 17). Retrieved from URL: https://draxe.com/l-glutamine-benefits-side-effects-dosage.

45. See above.

46. Healthline. *Top 6 Benefits of Taking Collagen Supplements.* Retrieved from URL: https://www.healthline.com/nutrition/collagen-benefits. See also Amy Myers, M.D. *Top 7 Health Benefits of Collagen & How to Get More*

47 Dr. Axe Food is Medicine. *Bone Broth Benefits for Digestion, Arthritis and Cellulite: Are They All They're Cracked up to Be?* (2019, January 23). Retrieved from URL: https://draxe.com/the-healing-power-of-bone-broth-for-digestion-arthritis-and-cellulite.

of It. Retrieved from URL: https://www.amymyersmd.com/2017/05/top-7-health-benefits-collagen-get.

48 The Guardian. *Can a Drink Really Make Skin Look Younger?* Retrieved from URL: https://www.theguardian.com/science/2015/sep/27/nutricosmetics-drink-make-skin-look-younger-science.

49 See above.

50 National Center for Biotechnology Information (NCBI) / PubMed.gov. *Glutamine enhances gut glutathione production.* (1998, July – August). Retrieved from URL: https://www.ncbi.nlm.nih.gov/pubmed/9661123?dopt=AbstractPlus. See also, *Perfect Health Diet* by Paul Jaminet, Ph.D. New York: Scribner Publishing, 2012. See also, Eat Beautiful. *GLUTAMINE: NOT Recommended for Leaky Gut.* Retrieved from URL: https://eatbeautiful.net/2015/12/28/glutamine-not-recommended-for-leaky-gut/.

51 ThoughtCo. *What Is Fermentation? Definition and Examples.* (2019, January 22). Retrieved from URL: https://www.thoughtco.com/what-is-fermentation-608199.

52 Chris Kesser. *Kefir: The Not-Quite-Paleo Superfood.* (2019, February 21). Retrieved from URL: https://chriskresser.com/kefir-the-not-quite-paleo-superfood.

53 Healthline. *9 Evidence-Based Health Benefits of Kefir.* Retrieved from URL: https://www.healthline.com/nutrition/9-health-benefits-of-kefir.

54 Academy of Nutrition and Dietetics. *Choose Healthy Fats.* (2019, February 6). Retrieved from URL: https://www.eatright.org/food/nutrition/dietary-guidelines-and-myplate/choose-healthy-fats.

55 See above.

56 Wellness Mama. *The Importance of Soaking Nuts & Seeds.* (2019, July 30). Retrieved from URL: https://wellnessmama.com/59139/soaking-nuts-seeds.

57 Egler, J., M.D. *7 Signs You Have a Hormone Imbalance.* Retrieved from URL: https://www.parsleyhealth.com/blog/hormonal-imbalance-symptoms.

58 See above.

59. Rawls MD. *The Hormone, Aging & Chronic Illness Connection*. Retrieved from URL: https://rawlsmd.com/health-articles/hormone-aging-chronic-illness-connection.
60. See above.
61. See above. See also, Siemens Healthineers. *Women and Autoimmune Disease*. Retrieved from URL: https://usa.healthcare.siemens.com/clinical-specialities/womens-health-information/laboratory-diagnostics/autoimmune-disorders.
62. See above.
63. Dr. K. News. *Hormonal imbalances? Estrogen clearance is vital to healthy hormone function*. Retrieved from URL: https://drknews.com/hormonal-imbalances-estrogen-clearance-vital-healthy-hormone-function.
64. John Hopkins Medicine. *Adrenal Glands*. Retrieved from URL: https://www.hopkinsmedicine.org/health/conditions-and-diseases/adrenal-glands.
65. *Adrenal Fatigue The 21st Century Stress Syndrome Wilson*, by James L. Wilson, N.D., D.C., Ph.D. Petaluma: Smart Publications, 2012.
66. See above, pp. 6-7.
67. See above.
68. Healthline. *12 Proven Benefits of Ashwagandha*. (2018, June 11). Retrieved from URL: https://www.healthline.com/nutrition/12-proven-ashwagandha-benefits.
69. See above.
70. Naturimedica. *Holy basil: a key herb for stress, anxiety, depression and fatigue*. Retrieved from URL: https://www.naturimedica.com/holy-basil-key-herb-stress-anxiety-depression-fatigue.
71. See above.
72. Floliving. *My Expert Opinion On Adaptogens For Hormone Health*. (2018, July 31). Retrieved from URL: https://www.floliving.com/adaptogens.
73. National Center for Biotechnology Information (NCBI). *Hormone Balancing Effect of Pre-Gelatinized Organic Maca*. (2006, September). Retrieved from URL: https://www.ncbi.nlm.nih.gov/pmc/articles/PMC3614604; See also, The Integrative Women's Health Institute. *Maca Powder Benefits ... Is Recommending Maca Good for Hormone Health or All Hype?* (2017, September 30). Retrieved from URL: https://integrativewomenshealthinstitute.com/is-adding-maca-to-your-smoothie

s-and-recommending-it-to-your-clients-a-good-idea-or-all-hype; See also, floliving. *My Expert Opinion on Adaptogens for Hormone Health.* (2018, July 31). Retrieved from URL: https://www.floliving.com/adaptogens.

74 Vital Plan. *Adaptogen Recovery.* Retrieved from URL: https://store.vitalplan.com/products/adaptogen-recovery.

75 Wellness Mama. *Ascorbic Acid: Vitamin C Benefits, Sources, & Cautions.* Retrieved from URL: https://wellnessmama.com/35500/vitamin-c-benefits. See also, National Center for Biotechnology Information (NCBI) / PubMed.gov. *Vitamin C is Important Cofactor for Both Adrenal Cortex and Adrenal Medulla.* (2004, November 30). Retrieved from URL: https://www.ncbi.nlm.nih.gov/pubmed/15666839. See also, The Adrenal Fatigue Solution. *Supplements for Adrenal Fatigue.* (2018, October 29). Retrieved from URL: https://adrenalfatiguesolution.com/adrenal-fatigue-supplements.

76 See above.

77 Mega Food. *Why Methylation Matters Part I.* Retrieved from URL: https://www.megafood.com/category/product-edu/methylation-matters-part-1-2.html.

78 Jacobs, J. Livestrong.com. *What Does Thytrophin PMG Do For Your Body?* Retrieved from URL: https://www.livestrong.com/article/484968-what-does-thytrophin-pmg-do-for-your-body.

79 WebMD. Thyroid Symptoms and Solutions. Retrieved from URL: https://www.webmd.com/women/ss/slideshow-thyroid-symptoms-and-solutions.

80 See above.

81 California Institute of Technology. *Microbes Help Produce Serotonin in Gut.* Retrieved from URL: http://www.caltech.edu/news/microbes-help-produce-serotonin-gut-46495.

82 MyDomaine. *From Mood to Mental Clarity, 7 Proven Ashwagandha Benefits.* (2019, May 29). Retrieved from URL: https://www.mydomaine.com/ashwagandha-benefits.

83 Healthline. *The Health Benefits of Holy Basil.* Retrieved from URL: https://www.healthline.com/health/food-nutrition/basil-benefits.

84 National Center for Biotechnology Information (NCBI) / PubMed.gov. *The Effect of Methylated Vitamin B Complex on Depressive and Anxiety Symptoms and Quality of Life in Adults with Depression.* (2013, January 21). Retrieved from URL: https://www.ncbi.nlm.nih.gov/pubmed/23738221.

85. Lara Briden—The Period Revolutionary. *The Curious Link Between Estrogen and Histamine Intolerance.* (2016, January 13). Retrieved from URL: https://www.larabriden.com/the-curious-link-between-estrogen-and-histamine-intolerance.
86. Amy Myers, M.D. *Everything You Need to Know About Histamine Intolerance.* Retrieved from URL: https://www.amymyersmd.com/2017/10/histamine-intolerance.
87. See above.
88. Vickery, A., Holistic Health Coach. *Histamine and Estrogen.* (2018, September 9). Retrieved from URL: https://alisonvickery.com.au/estrogen; see also, PubMed.gov. *Diamine oxidase (DAO) and female sex hormones.* (1986, April 18). Retrieved from URL: https://www.ncbi.nlm.nih.gov/pubmed/3088928; see also, Briden, L. (2016, January 13). *The Curious Link Between Estrogen and Histamine Intolerance.* Retrieved from URL: https://www.larabriden.com/the-curious-link-between-estrogen-and-histamine-intolerance.
89. See above.
90. Lara Briden—The Period Revolutionary. *The Curious Link Between Estrogen and Histamine Intolerance.* (2016, January 13). Retrieved from URL: https://www.larabriden.com/the-curious-link-between-estrogen-and-histamine-intolerance.
91. See above.
92. Vickery, A., Holistic Health Coach. *Histamine and Estrogen.* (2018, September 9). Retrieved from URL: https://alisonvickery.com.au/estrogen; see also, PubMed.gov. *Diamine oxidase (DAO) and female sex hormones.* (1986, April 18). Retrieved from URL: https://www.ncbi.nlm.nih.gov/pubmed/3088928; see also, Briden, L. (2016, January 13). *The Curious Link Between Estrogen and Histamine Intolerance.* Retrieved from URL: https://www.larabriden.com/the-curious-link-between-estrogen-and-histamine-intolerance.
93. Vickery, A., Holistic Health Coach. *Histamine and Estrogen.* (2018, September 9). Retrieved from URL: https://alisonvickery.com.au/estrogen; see also, PubMed.gov. *Diamine oxidase (DAO) and female sex hormones.* (1986, April 18). Retrieved from URL: https://www.ncbi.nlm.nih.gov/pubmed/3088928; see also, Briden, L. (2016, January 13). *The Curious Link Between Estrogen and Histamine Intolerance.* Retrieved

94   from URL: https://www.larabriden.com/the-curious-link-between-estrogen-and-histamine-intolerance.

94   Ingels, D., N.D. *5 Protocols for Treating Lyme Disease (and How to Tell Which is Right for You)*. (2018, April 5). Retrieved from URL: https://www.bewell.com/blog/5-protocols-for-treating-lyme-disease-and-how-to-tell-which-is-right-for-you.

95   Healthline. *6 Health Benefits of Apple Cider Vinegar, Backed by Science.* Retrieved from URL: https://www.healthline.com/nutrition/6-proven-health-benefits-of-apple-cider-vinegar.

96   Natural Living Ideas. *24 Baking Soda Uses & Why You Need It In Your Home.* (2014, September 24). Retrieved from URL: https://www.naturallivingideas.com/24-baking-soda-uses.

97   Science Daily. *Drinking Baking Soda Could Be an Inexpensive, Safe Way to Combat Autoimmune Disease.* (2018, April 25). Retrieved from URL: https://www.sciencedaily.com/releases/2018/04/180425093745.htm.

98   See above.

99   Jockers, D., D.N.M., D.C., M.S. *Using Baking Soda to Help Beat Cancer Naturally.* Retrieved from URL: https://drjockers.com/baking-soda-help-beat-cancer.

100   Metagenics. Retrieved from URL: https://www.metagenics.com/candibactin-ar.

101   Metagenics. Retrieved from URL: https://www.metagenics.com/candibactin-br.

102   Healthline. *Top 11 Science-Based Health Benefits of Pumpkin Seeds.* (2018, September 24). Retrieved from URL: https://www.healthline.com/nutrition/11-benefits-of-pumpkin-seeds#section1.

103   Juicing For Health. *How to Eat Pumpkin Seeds to Paralyze Parasites and Intestinal Worms for Elimination.* (2019, January 24). Retrieved from URL: https://juicing-for-health.com/pumpkin-seeds-paralyze-parasites-intestinal-worms.

104   See above.

105   See above.

106   Dr. Axe Food Is Medicine. *6 Proven Diatomaceous Earth Uses and Benefits.* (2018, November 2). Retrieved from URL: https://draxe.com/diatomaceous-earth. See also, Wellness Mama. *Diatomaceous Earth: 10*

Amazing Uses for DE Around the Home. (2019, January 23). Retrieved from URL: https://wellnessmama.com/13213/diatomaceous-earth.

107 See above.

108 Juicing For Health. *How to Eat Pumpkin Seeds to Paralyze Parasites and Intestinal Worms for Elimination.* (2019, January 24). Retrieved from URL: https://juicing-for-health.com/pumpkin-seeds-paralyze-parasites-intestinal-worms.

109 National Center for Biotechnology Information (NCBI) / PubMed.gov. *Small intestinal fungal overgrowth.* (2015, April 17). Retrieved from URL: https://www.ncbi.nlm.nih.gov/pubmed/25786900. See also, National Center for Biotechnology Information (NCBI) / PubMed.gov. *Small Intestinal Bacterial Overgrowth.* (2007, February 3). Retrieved from URL: https://www.ncbi.nlm.nih.gov/pmc/articles/PMC3099351. See also, Virgin, JJ. *How to Tell if You Have SIFO or SIBO.* Retrieved from URL: https://jjvirgin.com/are-you-sifo-sibo.

110 Body Ecology. *The Truth About Fermented Foods and SIBO.* Retrieved from URL: https://bodyecology.com/articles/the-truth-about-fermented-foods-and-sibo.

111 Virgin, JJ. *How to Tell if You Have SIFO or SIBO.* Retrieved from URL: https://jjvirgin.com/are-you-sifo-sibo.

112 Body Ecology. *The Low FODMAP Diet Warning for IBS and SIBO Sufferers.* Retrieved from URL: https://bodyecology.com/articles/the-low-fodmap-diet-warning-for-ibs-and-sibo-sufferers.

113 See above.

114 MedicineNet. *Low FODMAP Diet for IBS: List of Foods to Eat and Avoid.* Retrieved from URL: https://www.medicinenet.com/low_fodmap_diet_list_of_foods_to_eat_and_avoid/article.htm#fodmap_foods_for_ibs_definition_and_facts.

115 Body Ecology. *The Truth About Fermented Foods and SIBO.* Retrieved from URL: https://bodyecology.com/articles/the-truth-about-fermented-foods-and-sibo.

116 See above.

117 Natural On. *12 of the Best Anti-fungal Herbs on the Planet.* Retrieved from URL: https://naturalon.com/12-of-the-best-anti-fungal-herbs-on-the-planet/view-all.

[118] Wong, C., Very Well Health. *Natural Remedies for Bacterial Overgrowth.* (2018, November 17). Retrieved from URL: https://www.verywellhealth.com/natural-remedies-for-bacterial-overgrowth-89298.

[119] University Health News Daily. *SIBO Treatment with Herbs is as Effective as Anitbiotics.* (2018, June 29). Retrieved from URL: https://universityhealthnews.com/daily/digestive-health/sibo-treatment-with-herbs-is-as-effective-as-antibiotics-combine-with-a-sibo-diet-for-even-better-results.

[120] Bay Area Lyme Foundation. *Straight Talk About Biofilms: A New Answer for Treating Lyme Disease?* (2015, November 30). Retrieved from URL: https://www.bayarealyme.org/blog/straight-talk-biofilms-new-answer-treating-lyme-disease.

[121] LiveScience. *How Do Enzymes Work?* (2014, April 26). Retrieved from URL: https://www.livescience.com/45145-how-do-enzymes-work.html. See also, Global Health Center. *The Difference Between Systemic Enzymes and Digestive Enzymes.* (2018, June 19). Retrieved from URL: https://www.globalhealingcenter.com/natural-health/difference-systemic-enzymes-digestive-enzymes/

[122] See above.

[123] See above.

[124] LiveScience. *How Do Enzymes Work?* (2014, April 26). Retrieved from URL: https://www.livescience.com/45145-how-do-enzymes-work.html. See also, Global Health Center. *The Difference Between Systemic Enzymes and Digestive Enzymes.* (2018, June 19). Retrieved from URL: https://www.globalhealingcenter.com/natural-health/difference-systemic-enzymes-digestive-enzymes. See also, Nutrients for an Energetic Lifestyle. *Systemic Enzyme Therapy: Differences in Serrapeptase and Nattokinase.* (2017, February 14). Retrieved from URL: https://www.energeticnutrition.com/blog/2017/02/systemic-enzyme-therapy-differences-serrapeptase-nattokinase.

[125] PPT Health. *Fibrin in Bioflims and Cysts.* Retrieved from URL: https://www.ppt-health.com/lyme-disease-basics/fibrin-in-biofilms-and-cysts.

[126] LiveScience. *How Do Enzymes Work?* (2014, April 26). Retrieved from URL: https://www.livescience.com/45145-how-do-enzymes-work.html. See also, Global Health Center. *The Difference Between Systemic Enzymes and Digestive Enzymes.* (2018, June 19). Retrieved from

URL: https://www.globalhealingcenter.com/natural-health/difference-systemic-enzymes-digestive-enzymes. See also, Nutrients for an Energetic Lifestyle. *Systemic Enzyme Therapy: Differences in Serrapeptase and Nattokinase.* (2017, February 14). Retrieved from URL: https://www.energeticnutrition.com/blog/2017/02/systemic-enzyme-therapy-differences-serrapeptase-nattokinase.

127 See above.

128 See above.

129 See above.

130 Global Health Center. *The Difference Between Systemic Enzymes and Digestive Enzymes.* (2018, June 19). Retrieved from URL: https://www.globalhealingcenter.com/natural-health/difference-systemic-enzymes-digestive-enzymes.

131 See above.

132 ProHealth. *Cistus: A Natural Antibiotic, Antiviral, and Biofilm Buster.* (2016, July 28). Retrieved from URL: https://www.prohealth.com/library/cistus-a-natural-antibiotic-antiviral-and-biofilm-buster-6292.

133 Loomis Enzymes. *FARS-P.* Retrieved from URL: https://www.loomisenzymes.com/store/advanced/fars-p.aspx.

134 BiomedicLabsRx. *Dual Action Inflammation Support Bundles.* Retrieved from URL: https://www.biomediclabs.com/dual-action-inflammation-support-bundles.

135 See above.

136 Kresser, C. *What Everybody Ought to Know (But Doesn't) about Heartburn & GERD.* (2019, March 17). Retrieved from URL: https://chriskresser.com/what-everybody-ought-to-know-but-doesnt-about-heartburn-gerd.

137 See above.

138 See above.

139 See above.

140 MD Anderson Cancer Center. *Probiotics: Healthy Bacteria For Your Gut.* Retrieved from URL: https://www.mdanderson.org/publications/focused-on-health/FOH-probiotics.h14-1589835.html.

141 Medical News Today. *Chronic Fatigue Syndrome: Could Altered Gut Bacteria Be a Cause?* (2016, June 28). Retrieved from URL: https://www.medicalnewstoday.com/articles/311287.php.

142 Rhinehart, A., Master Healthy Living Coach. *Health Benefits of Bacillus Probiotics.* Retrieved from URL: https://info.dralexrinehart.com/articles/health-topics/immune-health/health-benefits-and-safety-bacillus-soil-based-spore-probiotics.

143 Microbiome Labs. *MegaSporeBiotic Spore Based Probiotic / Antioxidant.* Retrieved from URL: https://microbiomelabs.com/products/megasporebiotic.

144 US News & World Report. *What Are Prebiotics?* (2019, May 3). Retrieved from URL: https://health.usnews.com/health-news/blogs/eat-run/articles/what-are-prebiotics.

145 See above.

146 Healthline. *9 Evidence-Based Health Benefits of Kefir.* Retrieved from URL: https://www.healthline.com/nutrition/9-health-benefits-of-kefir.

147 See above.

148 Rawls MD. *Lyme + Herxheimer Reactions Your Guide to Feeling Good Again.* (2019, January 21). Retrieved from URL: https://rawlsmd.com/health-articles/lyme-herxheimer-reactions-your-guide-to-feeling-good-again.

149 Dr. Axe Food Is Medicine. *6 Proven Diatomaceous Earth Uses and Benefits.* (2018, November 2). Retrieved from URL: https://draxe.com/diatomaceous-earth. See also, Wellness Mama. *Diatomaceous Earth: 10 Amazing Uses for DE Around the Home.* (2019, January 23). Retrieved from URL: https://wellnessmama.com/13213/diatomaceous-earth.

150 See above.

151 National Center for Biotechnology Information (NCBI) / PubMed.gov. *The Neuroprotective Aspects of Sleep.* (2015, March 3). Retrieved from URL: https://www.ncbi.nlm.nih.gov/pmc/articles/PMC4651462. See also, National Center for Biotechnology Information (NCBI) / PubMed.gov. *Sleep facilitates clearance of metabolites from the brain; glymphatic function in aging and neurodegenerative diseases.* (2013, December 16). Retrieved from URL: https://www.ncbi.nlm.nih.gov/pubmed/24199995. See also, National Center for Biotechnology Information (NCBI) / PubMed.gov. *Amyloid-B diurnal pattern: possible role of sleep in Alzheimer's disease pathogenesis.* (2014, September). Retrieved from URL: https://www.ncbi.nlm.nih.gov/pubmed/24910393.

[152] Mark Hyman, M.D. *Functional Wellness, Part 6: Energy, Mitochondria and Toxicity.* (2008, December). Retrieved from URL: https://experiencelife.com/article/functional-wellness-part-6-energy-mitochondria-and-toxicity.

[153] See above.

[154] Johnston, B., Exercise Specialist, International Association of Resistance Training. *Benefits of Exercise.* Retrieved from URL: https://www.merckmanuals.com/home/fundamentals/exercise-and-fitness/benefits-of-exercise.

[155] See above.

[156] WebMD. *Ribose.* Retrieved from URL: https://www.webmd.com/vitamins-and-supplements/ribose-uses-and-risks#1. See also, VeryWellHealth. *D-Ribose for Fibromyalgia and Chronic Fatigue Syndrome.* (2018, December 4). Retrieved from URL: https://www.verywellhealth.com/d-ribose-for-fibromyalgia-715990.

[157] VeryWellHealth. *D-Ribose for Fibromyalgia and Chronic Fatigue Syndrome.* (2018, December 4). Retrieved from URL: https://www.verywellhealth.com/d-ribose-for-fibromyalgia-715990.

[158] See above.

[159] *100 Simple Things You Can Do to Prevent Alzheimer's*, by Jean Carper. New York: Hachette Book Group, 2012, pg. 18-20.

[160] See above.

[161] See above.

[162] See above.

[163] Healthline. *Top 9 Benefits of NAC (N-Acetyl Cysteine).* (2018, September 26). Retrieved from URL: https://www.healthline.com/nutrition/nac-benefits

[164] See above.

[165] Mark Hyman, M.D. *Essential Glutathione: The Mother of All Antioxidants.* Retrieved from URL: https://drhyman.com/blog/2010/05/19/glutathione-the-mother-of-all-antioxidants.

[166] Healthline. *Top 9 Benefits of NAC (N-Acetyl Cysteine).* (2018, September 26). Retrieved from URL: https://www.healthline.com/nutrition/nac-benefits.

[167] Healthline. *10 Evidence-Based Health Benefits of Magnesium.* (2018, September 3). Retrieved from URL: https://www.healthline.com/nutrition/10-proven-magnesium-benefits.

168 See above.

169 See above.

170 Medical News Today. *What Are the Benefits of CoQ10?* (2019, January 8). Retrieved from URL: https://www.medicalnewstoday.com/articles/324113.php.

171 See above.

172 National Center for Biotechnology Information (NCBI) / PubMed.gov. *Ubiquinol is Superior to Ubiquinone to Enhance Coenzyme Q10 Status in Older Men.* (2018, November 14). Retrieved from URL: https://www.ncbi.nlm.nih.gov/pubmed/30302465.

173 Medical News Today. *What Are the Benefits of CoQ10?* (2019, January 8). Retrieved from URL: https://www.medicalnewstoday.com/articles/324113.php.

174 Healthline. *11 Vitamins and Supplements that Boost Energy.* (2018, May 28). Retrieved from URL: https://www.healthline.com/nutrition/best-supplements-for-energy.

175 See above.

176 VeryWellHealth. *Creatine for Fibromyalgia and Chronic Fatigue Syndrome.* (2019, July 22). Retrieved from URL: https://www.verywellhealth.com/creatine-for-fibromyalgia-and-chronic-fatigue-syndrome-4149399.

177 Fox News. *Study Finds Traces of Drugs in Drinking Water in 24 Major US Regions.* (2008, March 10). Retrieved from URL: https://www.foxnews.com/story/study-finds-traces-of-drugs-in-drinking-water-in-24-major-u-s-regions.

178 See above.

179 See above.

180 ZeroWater. Retrieved from URL: https://www.zerowater.com.

181 See above.

182 See above.

183 The Berkey. Retrieved from URL: https://theberkey.com.

184 See above.

185 See above.

186 See above.

187 Berkley News. *Lotion Ingredient Paraben May Be More Potent Carcinogen Than Thought.* (2015, October 27). Retrieved from URL: https://news.berkeley.edu/2015/10/27/lotion-ingredient-paraben-may-be-more-potent-carcinogen-than-thought. See also, Scientific American. *Should People Be Concerned about Parabens in Beauty Products?* Retrieved

from URL: https://www.scientificamerican.com/article/should-people-be-concerned-about-parabens-in-beauty-products.

188 See above.
189 See above.
190 See above.
191 Berkley News. *Lotion Ingredient Paraben May Be More Potent Carcinogen Than Thought.* (2015, October 27). Retrieved from URL: https://news.berkeley.edu/2015/10/27/lotion-ingredient-paraben-may-be-more-potent-carcinogen-than-thought.
192 See above.
193 See above.
194 Well and Good. *Is Fluoride Actually Safe? Two Dentists Go Head to Head Over the Common Toothpaste Ingredient.* (2019, February 13). Retrieved from URL: https://www.wellandgood.com/good-advice/is-fluoride-healthy-and-safe
195 See above.
196 See above.
197 See above. See also, National Center for Biotechnology Information (NCBI) / PubMed.gov. *Aluminum and Alzheimer's Disease: After a Century of Controversy, Is There a Plausible Link?* Retrieved from URL: https://www.ncbi.nlm.nih.gov/pubmed/21157018.
198 International Academy of Oral Medicine & Toxicology. *Dental Amalgam Mercury Fillings and Danger to Human Health.* Retrieved from URL: https://iaomt.org/resources/dental-mercury-facts/amalgam-fillings-danger-human-health.
199 Pure Living Space. *Why You Should Avoid Toxic Dryer Sheets.* (2018, June 11). Retrieved from URL: https://purelivingspace.com/blogs/safe-laundry/why-you-should-avoid-toxic-dryer-sheets. See also, Dr. Axe Food Is Medicine. *Stop Using Dryer Sheets Immediately.* (2017, June 14). Retrieved from URL: https://draxe.com/dryer-sheets.
200 See above.
201 See above.
202 See above.
203 See above.
204 See above.
205 See above.

206 Silver Needle & Thread. *Frequently Used Toxic Chemicals In Your Clothes.* Retrieved from URL: http://www.silverneedleandthread.com/Chemicals-in-Clothes.html.

207 HuffPost. *Why You Should Watch Out for These Five Gnarly Chemicals in Your Clothing.* (2016, September 13). Retrieved from URL: https://www.huffpost.com/entry/these-are-the-gnarly-chemicals-in-the-cheap-clothes-we-buy_n_57d6e494e4b03d2d459b92ff.

208 See above.

209 See above.

210 See above.

211 See above.

212 Consumer Reports. *Wash and then Wear; Unwashed Clothes May Have Formaldehyde.* (2010, November 12). Retrieved from URL: https://www.consumerreports.org/cro/news/2010/11/wash-and-then-wear-unwashed-clothes-may-have-formaldehyde/index.htm.

213 HuffPost. *Why You Should Watch Out for These Five Gnarly Chemicals in Your Clothing.* (2016, September 13). Retrieved from URL: https://www.huffpost.com/entry/these-are-the-gnarly-chemicals-in-the-cheap-clothes-we-buy_n_57d6e494e4b03d2d459b92ff.

214 Environmental Working Group EWG. *Cleaning Supplies and Your Health.* Retrieved from URL: https://www.ewg.org/guides/cleaners/content/cleaners_and_health.

215 Environmental Working Group EWG. *EWG's Healthy Living Guide.* Retrieved from URL: https://www.ewg.org/healthyhomeguide/cleaners-and-air-fresheners/?gclid=Cj0KCQjwnpXmBRDUARIsAEo71tSo3OAJjHCFnpXSev8Blivp03DF7Sv7Th7QQS-p4_pPAvhoKaDBZdUaArHzEALw_wcB#.WmiqHlQ-eL4.

216 See above.

217 See above.

218 See above.

219 See above.

220 See above.

221 See above.

222 Time. *You Asked: Is My Air Conditioner Killing Me?* (2015, July 1). Retrieved from URL: http://time.com/3942050/air-conditioner-healthy.

223 Wellness Mama. *Is EMF Exposure Really a Big Deal?* (2019, January 9). Retrieved from URL: https://wellnessmama.com/129645/emf-exposure. See also, Defender Shield. *How Airplane Mode Helps Reduce*

Your EMF Radiation Exposure. (2018, December 17). Retrieved from URL: https://www.defendershield.com/how-airplane-mode-helps-reduce-your-emf-radiation-exposure.

[224] See above.

[225] See above.

[226] See above.

[227] Organic Authority. *8 Non-Toxic Cookware Brands to Keep Chemicals Out of Your Food.* (2019, May 7). Retrieved from URL: https://www.organicauthority.com/organic-food-recipes/non-toxic-cookware-brands-to-keep-chemicals-out-of-your-food.

[228] See above.

[229] See above. See also, National Center for Biotechnology Information (NCBI) / PubMed.gov. *Aluminum and Alzheimer's Disease: After a Century of Controversy, Is There a Plausible Link?* Retrieved from URL: https://www.ncbi.nlm.nih.gov/pubmed/21157018.

Printed in Great Britain
by Amazon